D0458800

is it **me**

or my **meds**?

is it **me**
or my **meds**?

WITHDRAWN

Living with

Antidepressants

David A. Karp

HARVARD UNIVERSITY PRESS

Cambridge, Massachusetts

London, England

2006

Printed in the United States of America

Many of the designations used by manufacturers and sellers to
distinguish their products are claimed as trademarks. Where
those designations appear in this book and Harvard University
Press was aware of a trademark claim, then the designations
have been printed in initial capital letters (for example, Prozac).

Library of Congress Cataloging-in-Publication Data

Karp, David Allen, 1944–
   Is it me or my meds? : living with antidepressants / David A.
Karp.
      p.   cm.
   Includes bibliographical references and index.
   ISBN 0-674-02182-7 (alk. paper)
   1. Antidepressants—Anecdotes.   2. Depressed persons—
Anecdotes.   3. Depression, Mental—Chemotherapy—
Anecdotes.   I. Title.

RC537.K3665 2006
616.85′27061—dc22   2006041061

To Darleen

My wife, my best friend, and my collaborator
in all the important things

Contents

is it **me**

or my **meds**?

Prologue: Doxepin Diary

I'm reaching the point where I will do anything for a good night's sleep. I truly feel desperate. I get applause from family and friends about hanging in there, but I'm not feeling terribly courageous and brave right now. . . . I'm monitoring my feelings from moment to moment and it seems so endless. I feel as though I will never be well. . . . I'm just about off the drugs and probably as miserable as I have ever been in my life.

—"Doxepin Diary,"
July 22, 2001

In the summer of 2001 I undertook a personally important life experiment. For the first time in a decade, I swallowed less than 100 milligrams of doxepin at bedtime. I had often imagined what life would be like without psychiatric drugs—the doxepin, Klonopin, and self-prescribed melatonin I had been taking every night. At age fifty-seven I wondered just who I might be if I were free of medications. After all, I was surely not the same person who embarked on a drug career at age thirty-one. But in the past I had always given myself some reason for not making the change: "I can't afford to experiment with important family events approaching." "If things go badly I'll never finish my research." "Not now, just before our trip to Africa." "I can't make a change at the beginning of a new semester." At last, driven by a range of motives, I committed the summer of 2001 to tapering off psychotropic drugs.

One important moment in my evolving drug consciousness came at a symposium in Chicago. The daylong meeting was devoted to the connections among illnesses, medications, and identities. Speakers from a variety of disciplines—anthropologists, sociologists, pharmacists, and psychiatrists—were brought together to discuss the intersections of health and the "self." Spending the day talking to bright people with a critical edge to their thinking about drugs, pharmaceutical companies, and identity was greatly instructive. My new colleagues taught me that most pharmacists, internists, and psychiatrists rarely think about the impact of medications on anything other than the body's cells. As a social psychologist, habitually drawn to issues of meaning and identity, I was stunned by such conceptual myopia.

The actual decision to get off antidepressants was made abruptly. I had not seen a psychiatrist for several months. I was overdue: psychiatrists are ordinarily expected to meet with their drug-taking patients at least twice a year. A few hours before my appointment, with the conversation at the symposium fresh in my mind, I decided to tell my doctor (I'll call him Bob) that I wanted to stop my medications. I'd seen Bob only twice. My previous psychiatrist could no longer see me, and I'd simply been assigned to Bob. I did like Bob, though, and I felt reasonably comfortable talking with him even though his sensibilities did not seem to include my sociological angle of vision. Bob believed unambiguously in biology.

Every time I tried to gain clarity on precisely why I felt I should stop the drugs, I got stuck. I now realize that I was driven as much by emotion as by any rational assessment of what would be a good course of action for a middle-aged man with a long history of depression and anxiety. I continue to ask myself these kinds of questions: Should I be so dependent on pills? Are drugs for diabetes really comparable to those for depression, or is that just another tactic to pathologize bad feelings? Why am I not equally worried about nonpsychiatric medications? Do psychotropic medications shape my identity? Then again, what's the big deal about taking a few pills each night? I've been doing it for so long now. Why shouldn't I just keep using them for the rest of my life? And yet, perhaps the drugs themselves are responsible for the many awful days and nights I've experienced over the years. There have been so many days when I've felt "drugged."

My discomfort with psychiatry has accelerated in recent years. After one Friday night dinner, my wife and I took a brief tour of a local bookstore, as we often do. A book by the Harvard psychiatrist Joseph Glenmullen caught my eye. Its title: *Prozac Backlash: Overcoming the Dangers of Prozac, Zoloft, Paxil, and Other Antidepressants with Safe, Effective Alternatives.* I had read works like this before and they had always upset me—books like Peter Breggin's *Toxic Psychiatry* or Stephen Fried's *Bitter Pills.* Reading Glenmullen was rather like a continuation of the conversation at the Chicago Symposium, except even more troubling. The problem with new psychiatric drugs, he said, is that their effects are sometimes not clear for ten, twenty, or thirty years. Because Prozac-type drugs have been around only since the early 1980s, millions of patients don't know about the potential dangers of SSRIs (selective serotonin reuptake inhibitors). Citing studies and his own clinical experience, Glenmullen detailed the emerging and unsettling long-term effects of these drugs. At one point he offered the unhappy thought that 150 years from now future generations may look back on the anti-depressant era as a frightening experiment.

I never know quite how to respond to books like Breggin's, Glenmullen's, or Fried's. Are these guys simply alarmist ideologues, as their critics claim? Don't all drugs have problems? Certainly, despite their side effects, we wouldn't throw away the hundreds of drugs that clearly improve people's lives. Medicine always operates in terms of a risk/reward ratio when it evaluates drugs. Of course, it's easy to be cool and rational about such ratios when you're a researcher studying drugs or a doctor assessing the best treatment for a patient. It's quite another thing to be the patient dealing with real-life drug trials.

Tapering off doxepin and Klonopin was not fun. For the first few weeks I did pretty well. Although I noticed an increase in my usual morning anxiety, it was nothing especially alarming. But when I finally reached one-fourth of my normal dose, I got very sick. My sleeping, always the barometer of my emotional well-being, eroded badly. I documented this process in my "Doxepin Diary":

Thursday, June 7, 12:20 P.M.

I just dragged myself out of bed. What a night! I'm
sure I slept some after writing in this journal until
4:30 A.M. But it was not the kind of sleep anyone
would want. It certainly wasn't a dream of peace. My
waking time was a combination of feeling bone tired
while my head whirled with agitation. It was not anxiety in the pure form that I sometimes know it. It was
more of a spinning sense as though my brain would
not shut off. When I did fall asleep my fate was to
dream vivid and disturbing dreams. I can't remember
their content but I do remember having several. They
weren't precisely of the nightmare variety, but they
felt distressing. Right now I'm drinking a cup of cof-
fee with the hope that the pressure on the top of my
head will subside. It's unpredictable what becomes of
the pressure during the day. Sometimes, if I'm lucky,
it wears off the way that the morning fog over San
Francisco Bay sometimes gives way to clarity and sun.
On other days, the brain fog lingers all day, casting a
mental pall over every activity.

Sunday, June 17, 10:45 A.M.

Last night I hoped that my exhaustion would save me
from insomnia. Unhappily, I had my third sleepless
night in a row. The night was its usual horror. I
loathe the middle of the night when my brain and
my emotions are in such turmoil. I feel the most fran-
tic in the middle of the night when I can't sleep. I
hate these nights so profoundly. I feel in danger of

going crazy at 3 or 4 A.M. This is when I am the most
vulnerable. In the middle of a sleepless night my ob-
sessions kick into overdrive. I feel that maybe I be-
long in a hospital.

Monday, June 25, 9:30 A.M.
I'm foggy again. I'd like to move ahead with some
writing on drugs beyond the notes I'm keeping here. I
just don't think I have enough mental clarity to do
that. It feels like it's a huge task just to get these
words down. Everything feels so effortful when your
head is clogged and you feel sleep deprived. It doesn't
feel like you're alive. I've had some truly "dead days"
in my life and I'm not at that point right now. I'm
somewhere between dead and alive. Depression
limbo. Drug limbo. Life limbo.

Throughout this time I vacillated, often within minutes and throughout the days and nights, about the wisdom of my decision to stop taking medication. I could
not distinguish the effects of stopping the drugs from a
ferocious return of my mental illness. My resolve to complete the experiment was most severely tested and ultimately dissolved by social obligations, especially those involving travel and "good times."

The breaking point came in August. My daughter and
her husband were preparing to leave for Senegal for two
years on a project to diminish conflict between the government and a rebel movement. My wife and I decided to
spend a weekend with them in Las Vegas before their de-

parture. After several nights of almost no sleep, I felt tormented by the journey , saved only by the fact that I could withdraw into the airplane seat and into myself. Once in Las Vegas, everyone wanted to go out on the town. I was frozen by fatigue, anxiety, and sadness and simply could not face the lights, the movement, and the jangling sounds. I refused to leave the room. At that moment I knew my decision to stop the medication had failed, and I took some Klonopin. That night, I slept better than I had in weeks. The relief was enormous.

Let me briefly bring you up to date on my awkward dance with medications. I discovered that stopping Klonopin was far more difficult than I had imagined. I had slowly tapered the dose over a period of three months. After my relapse in Las Vegas I made a full return to Klonopin; in fact, I now take twice the previous dose. Rather like the face-saving claims of the United States in Vietnam, I surrendered to the Klonopin while declaring victory. At least I was no longer taking doxepin. I've since learned that stopping benzodiazepines like Klonopin, Valium, and Xanax is not easy since many patients become habituated to these drugs.

Even my partial victory, cutting down from two drugs to one, was short-lived. At Bob's suggestion, I agreed to take trazodone, a drug I had taken unsuccessfully in the 1980s. Trazodone, he explained, is the antidepressant workhorse for sleep. It did help, but my sleeping was still unsound. Each time I met with Bob he gently urged me to try an SSRI. He expressed confidence that Celexa would reduce my worry and improve my sleep. After a second opinion concurred with Bob's hopeful scenario, I decided to give it a try.

Just as Bob predicted, things dramatically improved after a few weeks. I felt reborn and approached each day with an enthusiasm that I had forgotten was possible. But after another few weeks I began to have bad days and nights; moreover, I learned that I was among the approximately 50 percent of patients whose sexuality is affected by SSRIs. Bob suggested adding Wellbutrin or even Ritalin to my cocktail of Celexa, Klonopin, and trazodone. I was unwilling, though, to add drugs to fix a drug-induced problem. At this writing I am unsuccessfully experimenting with smaller doses of Celexa and am strongly considering stopping it altogether.

Like most of the people whose voices you will hear in this book, I am on an uncertain journey. It is easy to get horribly lost. There are no maps. You're driving on dimly lit and poorly marked roads that require constant guesses about which turns to take. Unsettling detours are the norm. The trip is exhausting and you never quite know how far you have traveled. You hope to get to a healthy place, but you're not sure where it is, whether you'll ever arrive, or even whether that destination exists for you.

Chapter 1

Giving Voice

The voices of the ill are easy to ignore, because these voices are often faltering in tone and mixed in message. . . . These voices bespeak conditions . . . that most of us would rather forget our vulnerability to. Listening is hard, but it is also a fundamentally moral act. . . . In listening for the other, we listen for ourselves. The moment of witness in the story crystallizes a mutuality of need, when each is for the other.

—Arthur Frank, *The Wounded*
Storyteller, p. 25

I have simple writing goals. I listen to people's stories about aspects of their lives that matter greatly to them. Then I try to convey those stories—those gifts, really—as faithfully as possible. Of course, I also try to see patterns in the accounts I hear and to place stories within a larger framework in order to make sense of commonalties. However, in all of this I keep one thing very clearly in mind: while I may have some insights to share from listening carefully and thinking theoretically, I am not the expert. I approach people to interview in the first place because they share a life circumstance that I want to know more about. They themselves are the experts; I have the privilege of learning from them.

Here I give fifty people with a diagnosed mental illness a platform for describing their experiences with psychiatric drugs.[1] Emotionally ill people and their families rarely get to speak their minds in public discourse about their illness. Rather, most of our information on these matters comes from professional experts. While doctors, nurses, social workers, psychologists, sociologists, and an assortment of therapists bring useful academic and clinical perspectives to issues surrounding mental health, their efforts typically bypass the stories of ill people themselves. A number of memoirists have described lives bounded by mental illness and often, therefore, by mind-altering pills.[2] Although these accounts provide eloquent, insightful testimony on the complexity of living with a stigmatized illness, each book is limited by its author's particular biography. This book, in contrast, will be organized around the central, repeating, and common dimensions of psychotropic drug use that become discernible only when one listens to a variety of personal narratives focused explicitly on that subject.

I offered a piece of my own story in the Prologue to let you know my biases, and to illustrate the kind of ambivalence that often accompanies pill-taking. My experiences also frame the way I make sense of what my interviewees say. I agree with the sociologist Susan Krieger that "when we discuss others, we are always talking about ourselves."[3] At the same time, my interpretations are disciplined by carefully collected data, in this case by the narratives I have gathered. Despite my own critical attitude toward the drugs I take, my intention is not to debunk psychiatry or to resolve whether current biological theories of mental illness are correct. Rather, my aim is to understand the experience of taking psychiatric medications *from the point of view of patients*. Arthur Kleinman, a psychiatrist and anthropologist, has it right when he observes:

> Social reality is so organized that we do not routinely inquire into the meanings of illness any more than we regularly analyze the structure of our social world. Indeed, the everyday priority structure of medical training and of health care delivery, with its radically materialist pursuit of the biological mechanism of disease, precludes such inquiry. It turns the gaze of the clinician, along with the attention of patients, away from decoding the salient meanings of illness for them. . . . The biomedical system replaces this allegedly "soft," therefore devalued, psychosocial concern with meanings with the scientifically "hard," therefore overvalued, technical quest for the control of symptoms. This pernicious value transformation is a serious failing of modern medicine; it disables the healer and disempowers the chronically ill.[4]

I want the narratives in this book to enable healers and to empower patients. Those who practice the healing arts need to recognize that human beings are not inanimate receptacles for medical treatments. Rather, patients seek to give meaning to and impose order on their illnesses. Consequently, the decision to use psychiatric drugs is rarely made unthinkingly. Visiting a doctor and then filling a prescription for antidepressants is normally a weighty affair, bounded by ongoing and extensive interpretations about the nature of one's pain, about mental illness, and about medical expertise. Equally, the meanings attached to psychotropic medications shift over time as people try to sort out just how well the drugs are working.

All drugs, legal or illegal, require people to continually justify their use and evaluate their consequences. Certainly, every drug has the potential to affect mood and cognition. Blood pressure medications, for example, can alter emotions and perceptions. Sometimes unintended effects are so unpleasant that people decide to stop using the drugs. However, I maintain that psychiatric medications are qualitatively different from other medications. The important point here is that, in contrast to other medications, *psychotropic drugs have as their purpose the transformation of people's moods, feelings, and perceptions.* These drugs act on—perhaps even create—people's consciousness and, therefore, have profound effects on the nature of their identities.

I remember pondering questions of self the first time I read Peter Kramer's book *Listening to Prozac.*[5] Some of the stories Kramer tells are both miraculous and disturbing. For instance, he describes a woman, once so incapacitated by social anxiety that she rarely left home, who became a social butterfly after boosting her serotonin level via

Prozac. If people can change so dramatically by altering even slightly the volume of neurotransmitters in their brains, we need to wonder just who we are and what exactly makes us human. Consequently, people's attitudes and feelings about psychiatric medications go well beyond questions of health and illness. These drugs often cause people to confront basic issues about their own humanity. In particular, we need to ask why medications that sometimes dramatically relieve human suffering make some people uncomfortable with their new, "healthier" selves.[6]

Although people are often skittish about taking *any* new and powerful medication, the decision to take psychiatric drugs can be particularly difficult. Some patients worry about how the drugs might harm their bodies and minds. Most also fear that their identities might be altered. One person expressed it this way: "I didn't think I needed [the medication]. I didn't like being considered depressed. I felt like Zoloft was for people who were really depressed and I . . . didn't feel like I fit in that category." For most people the decision to start taking psychiatric drugs marks a significant change in the way they see their illness. More profoundly, taking the pills initiates a potentially life-altering process of self-transformation. For many, psychotropic drugs provoke some basic questions: Who am I? How have I become the person I am? To what degree am *I* in control of my emotions, thoughts, and perceptions?

In her memoir *Prozac Diary*, Lauren Slater describes how Prozac liberated her from debilitating depression and a crippling obsessive compulsive disorder. For her, the pills carried magical, even religious significance. Yet she grappled with whether to keep taking the drug. The interesting question is why she and others routinely entertain the idea of stopping medications that have freed them from such terrible pain. In Slater's case the drug, while diminishing her torment, also made her indifferent to writing, previously her passion. The anxiety-driven urge to self-expression by which she had always defined herself was blunted, nearly eradicated. When she complained to her doctor about not feeling her "self," though her worst obsessive-compulsive symptoms had virtually disappeared, he first suggested upping the dose:

> He told me to take two capsules a day instead of one, which, at first, I didn't do. In fact, I was thinking about stopping the Prozac altogether, torn between my desire for my old self and my enthusiasm for the new. I was concerned that Prozac, and the health it spawned, could take away not only my creativity but my very identity. . . . I was a different person now, both more and less like me, fulfilling one possibility while swerving from another. There is loss in that swerving. And my experience on Prozac showed me how few there are who understand that loss or are prepared for its expression.[7]

Toward the end of the book Slater returns to the same themes:

Given my questions, maybe it would be wiser if I stopped the drug. Actually, I have tried several times. I decrease my dose slowly, inching down day by day, and then I cease altogether. Or I forget to take my dose one day, and then again the next, and by the time I have remembered I think, *What the hell, let's see what happens.* I picture myself drug-free, managing my life, and I get a jolt of joy. Sometimes, in the movie theater or the supermarket, I look around at people who I suppose live their lives without a chemical crutch, and they amaze me. There is a woman with a yellow scarf knotted around her neck. The yellow is the color of corn, of sunflowers, and she herself seems to have sprung from the garden. There are the children on the street. *To live without a drug.* After so many years, that to me is like living without water, something I cannot imagine, and the people who do this have a certain stature in my eyes.[8]

It would be a real stretch to say that psychotropic drugs provoke all users to muse about consciousness, identity, and self. The sociologist Philip Rieff once suggested that a "therapeutic state" had triumphed in America.[9] Along with Rieff and others, I'm prone to argue that a necessary condition for widespread psychiatric drug use is a culturally induced readiness to view emotional pain as a disease requiring medical intervention. With the growth of the therapeutic professions and the efforts of pharmaceutical companies to market solutions for every imaginable discomfort, the line between normal life pain and genuine pathology has become seriously blurred. The effort to secure personal happiness has become a social mandate, if not a moral obligation.[10] Consequently, many Americans consider psychotropic drug use perfectly "natural"; it has simply become a way of life.

With such issues in mind I talked with people who were being treated with medications for either depression or manic depression. Initially, I recruited several of my interviewees through my membership in an organization called MDDA—The Manic-Depressive and Depressive Association. I have attended MDDA's weekly "sharing and caring" support groups with some regularity for about fifteen years. The stories I hear in this forum astonish me by their poignancy, courage, and drama. Almost invariably, the accounts turn to the efficacy and meaning of medications. Although most people acknowledge that the drugs prevent their worst "episodes," they also express distress about the ways the medications affect their bodies and minds.

Mental illness displays itself in a wide variety of shades and intensities. Along with those whose day-to-day functioning is so severely impaired that they are unable to work or easily maintain conventional social ties are many people whose daily lives have at least the appearance of normality. These folks suffer from diseases severe enough to warrant diagnosis and medical treatment but hold onto jobs and fulfill most of their social obligations. Although I tried to speak to a range of ill people for this book, from the "walking wounded" to those who have been flattened by affective disorders, my sample is skewed toward those who are more severely ill than would be the case for all Americans treated with psychiatric medications. Eighteen of the forty adults and four of the ten children with whom I spoke have been sufficiently ill to spend time in hospitals. The patterns I describe cut across levels of illness severity, but I suspect that the identity issues at the core of my analyses are most cogently felt by people whose lives have been most deeply touched by mental illness.[11]

Too much of the current discussion about the use and efficacy of psychiatric drugs proceeds from extreme, often ideologically based positions. Writers like Harold Koplewicz and Samuel Barondes tout the new categories of antidepressants as offering dramatic help for depression and other mood disorders.[12] Others maintain that beyond their status as false saviors, psychiatric drugs are downright dangerous. Drawing inspiration from an earlier generation of social scientists who insisted that mental illness is nothing more than a politically inspired label for nonconforming behavior, writers like Peter Breggin keep telling Americans that "drugs might be your worst problem" and that psychopharmacologists are practicing "toxic psychiatry." To balance the picture we must learn how psychiatric patients themselves—the real experts in their drama—try to make sense of what their prescribed medications do to them and for them.[13]

Throughout this book I will keep returning to a number of fundamental drug-related questions that persist during the course of people's drug careers. The initial and most fundamental question for them is "Must I take drugs for my pain?" Once people begin taking medications for depression or manic depression, they are confronted by a host of additional questions: How well are the drugs working? Are the side effects bearable? Might other drugs or other doses work better? Will drugs ever solve my problem? How much do medical experts really know? Should I stop taking my medication? Who am I when I take mind-altering medications?

As with all important life questions, these cannot be answered once and for all. The meanings attached to medications change over the course of their use. Still, the inevitable efforts to answer such questions mirror the problematic and elusive character of drug-taking itself. Thus, a central task of this book is to illuminate how people grope toward tentative and workable answers to questions that cut to the core of illness and emotional pain, and so to the character of our very humanness.

Chapter 2

Unwelcome Careers

I know I'm better on medication . . . [but] there's been a persistent confusion about the real me since I started taking Prozac.

—Rachel, accountant,

aged 29

I'm no longer . . . thinking that there is something around the corner that I can try and that's going to give me a normal life. . . . I put myself in the category of treatment resistant after a while.

—Mike, unemployed, aged 51

Just like they said, after about five weeks I was feeling fantastic. I was back to like my normal self. I was feeling super. Yeah, I felt really great. And I said, "These drugs are great."

—Emily, educational

administrator, aged 51

To judge from the television advertisements touting their effectiveness, antidepressants would seem virtually infallible. Such ads usually begin with a woman (rarely a man) whose demeanor suggests considerable mental pain. Then, we are informed that if we have had the requisite number of symptoms (listed for our benefit) for at least two consecutive weeks, we may be suffering from depression (a diagnosis that must, of course, be verified by our family physician). Since some explanation of how the medicines work is called for, we are told that depression is caused by a chemical imbalance in the brain that can be corrected by the medication. The advertisement ends with the formerly pained woman now surrounded by her husband and children, smiling widely, and engaged in some high-energy activity. Before running off she may look directly into the camera to tell us that she now has her life back.

I have spent hundreds of hours listening to people in a support group talk about medications. Although the organization that runs the group prefers that members not offer advice about medications, many of the conversations begin with someone expressing confusion about the drugs he or she is taking or will shortly begin taking. Members then share their experiences with the same medication. During one such conversation, someone suggested that the medications work in one of three ways. First, they do exactly what they are supposed to do. Second, they don't do much of anything. Third, they do the opposite of what is expected. On the basis of my personal experience, as well as years spent listening to people talk about their struggles with medications, including the interviews done for this book, I am convinced that the caustic comment of my support group colleague gets us far closer to the truth than do drug advertisements.

In this chapter I will present the accounts of three of my interviewees, whose stories illustrate three broad and persistent patterns of response to psychotropic drugs. Naturally, it is problematic to generalize from three cases; after all, no two individuals face precisely the same contingencies as they try to work out the puzzles generated by their illness and the medications prescribed for it. Nonetheless, these cases preview my thinking in later chapters about commonalties in people's thoughts, feelings, and actions toward medications.

The account I heard most often in my interviews mirrors my own experience. It is one of ambivalence toward medications, of reluctance to rely on them, of movement from one drug or dose to another, and of uncertainty about the treatment's efficacy. It also hints at the process through which a clear majority of patients move—from initial resistance to a grudging acceptance of their need for medication. Eventually, those who follow this archetypal career capitulate to the idea that they will probably have to take medication for the rest of their lives. The first narrative, then, is one of partial success. We will hear it from Rachel, a twenty-nine-year-old accountant, whose depression was severe enough to have included a suicide attempt at age eighteen.

A second trajectory describes those who are, according to physicians, "treatment resistant." Mike, fifty-one years old and unemployed, described depression so severe that "it has just trashed my life." Although his articulate, often eloquent words revealed a lively and acute mind, no medication among the dozens he had tried ever gave him enough sustained respite from illness to realize his considerable potential. Now, after decades of disappointment, he is reconciled to a lifelong struggle with mental illness. Still, his story reveals the kind of courage required to keep trying in the face of a debilitating and unforgiving illness that current medicines cannot tame.

For a third, smaller group of those I interviewed, psychiatric medications worked like magic. Emily, a fifty-one-year-old educational administrator, suffered two incapacitating episodes of anxiety and depression following crises in her physical health. Gripped by a fear of death after a hysterectomy, Emily retreated to bed suffering from physical pains that she described as worse than childbirth. Because she was unable to eat, her weight plummeted dangerously, and her fear of death was replaced by the feeling that she might be better off dead. Initially, her pain was exacerbated by unsympathetic doctors and family members who minimized her symptoms and urged her to "pull herself together." Eventually a diagnosis of depression led her to Prozac and total cure of her symptoms, precisely in the time frame predicted by a psychiatric nurse. Although she later had to deal with multiple doctors and medications to combat troubling side effects, Emily nevertheless felt nearly undiluted enthusiasm for medications that, she said, "have saved me."

Rocks and Hard Places

Although the gap appears to be closing, the rate of depression among women is nearly twice that of men.[1] I find it very unlikely that women are somehow more vulnerable to depression because of the hard-wiring of their brains. I'm more inclined to suspect that social roles and cultural expectations increase women's vulnerability to a number of emotional disorders. One line of thinking has it that depression becomes more probable when people persistently feel obliged to repress and mute their thoughts and feelings, when there is, as Dana Jack has put it, a "silencing of the self."[2]

Rachel's account is partly the story of a young woman's efforts to discover her own authentic voice. One of my first questions in our conversation was "Where is home?" She replied, "I don't think I have a home." Rachel's response became less puzzling when she later described growing up in a family dominated by a mother's mental illness and a father's physical abuse, a circumstance tailor-made to stifle a young girl's selfhood. Such an outcome may be heightened for a child who takes on the role of "family peacekeeper." Here is how Rachel depicted her family life and relationships:

> My mother is mentally ill. She's never been diagnosed, she's never sought treatment. She doesn't even go to the doctor for normal routine visits. But she would do things . . . like when my parents would fight she would keep my father up for days at a time. Every

time he would try to go to sleep she would just yell at
him and pick at him and torture him so he couldn't
sleep. She would do things like take the largest knife
she could find in the kitchen and drive somewhere
and call the house and say, "You have fifteen minutes
to find me or I'll be dead." She once held a knife to
my throat for about twenty-four hours. Because I was
Daddy's favorite, the way to hurt Dad was to hurt
me. My role in all of that is that I was the peacekeeper. . . . I am the youngest. I have an older brother
and an older sister. My brother is five years older than
me and my sister is just a year older than me. When
my parents fought, my father would eventually get to
the point where he would hit my mother, and if my
brother got in between them, he would hit my
brother. If my sister got in between them, he would
hit my sister. And if I got in between them, he would
turn and walk away. Until I was about sixteen, he
never touched me. . . . As far as my mother was concerned she had a lot of resentment toward me because he wouldn't touch me.

Rachel said she had been depressed "for as long as I can
remember." Throughout elementary, middle, and high
school, "I spent a lot of time crying, a lot of time by myself. . . . As I got older I cried less but spent more time
alone. I was happier alone." Part of self-silencing is becoming skilled at putting on social performances at odds
with one's real feelings.[3] Rachel was "very good at giving a
show": "My father called me his little sunshine, and he

was very upset when I was first diagnosed with depression because that's not the way he sees me. He sees me very different from who I really am." She added: "I thought everyone was performing when I was very young."

By the time she got to high school, Rachel could no longer mask her depression and, like other young people with whom I have spoken, "started making some friends who were also depressed." These friends were a "lifeline," Rachel told me: "There were times when I really wanted to kill myself [and] they were the ones who stopped me." As a preventive measure Rachel made a pact with a fellow sufferer, Alex, "that neither of us would kill ourselves without the other one." At Alex's urging, she went to see the school counselors:

> I leveled with them. I told them that I cried a lot, that I would rather be alone than with people, and that really the only people that mattered to me were my friends who were depressed like me. At the time I was cutting myself also. I would go in and proudly show [the cutting] . . . [as if] to say, "I'm unhappy . . . look at how unhappy I am."

The cutting allowed Rachel to access feelings that she had long shut off:

> It served two functions. And I did cutting and burning. The burning came later when I was in college. I had the tendency to become very numb, to get to the point where I felt nothing because I was so sick of

hurting that I would just turn everything off. And
the cutting and burning was a way to . . . let that pain
out. That was why I was bulimic, too. Throwing up
for me was my way of getting anger out. If I couldn't
throw up I couldn't express any anger. And the cutting and burning, it was a way of me letting my pain
out and it was a way of me showing people, "Yeah,
I'm in pain."

The school counselors, appropriately alarmed by Rachel's account, referred her to a doctor who immediately
put her on drugs. The doctor's decision did not come as a
surprise: "I knew it was coming because I had friends in
similar situations and because they had recently been put
on medication. . . . And at first I welcomed it. I thought I
could take a pill and I would be normal. I would be fine. I
thought it was great. Yeah, you take a pill. Everything's
better. It's all sunshine and rainbows." Instead Rachel
discovered, to her dismay, that the combination of nortriptyline and trazodone only caused *more* numbness: "I
went from crying all the time and feeling sad all the time
to just not feeling anything." When I asked her which was
worse, the depression or the numbness, she said:

That's a tough question. . . . Being numb is easier, I
think, than being sad and depressed all the time, but
I think it's . . . much more dangerous. I stopped caring about everything. I stopped caring about life. I
stopped caring about whether I woke up in the
morning. I stopped caring about just everything.

Through her last three years of high school Rachel suffered from terrible insomnia: "Even on the medication, I didn't sleep more than two hours a night. . . . I mean, my nails were a different color each day of the week. . . . I would sit up at night and polish my nails for whatever outfit I was wearing the next day." Somehow she got through high school and made her way to college, where she requested a single room, telling school officials that she "was an insomniac and couldn't stand to watch someone else sleeping." While such self-imposed isolation provides short-term comfort, it is the crucible for greater long-term suffering. As people retreat from human connections, the necessary foundation for a viable self is compromised, the social world appears still more forbidding, and the urge to withdraw, in turn, further intensifies. Though Rachel had hoped that leaving for college would liberate her from her depression, in fact the downward spiral of hopelessness, withdrawal, and erosion of self led her to attempt suicide after her freshman year.

Once Rachel was hospitalized the doctors put her on Prozac. The trial of Prozac was short, however, because it made her so sick to her stomach. The replacement, Wellbutrin, was even worse: it threw her into anaphylactic shock. Shortly after taking the medication she noticed hives on her body. A nurse dismissed the symptom, insisting that it could not be caused by the medication. But Rachel woke up the next morning covered with hives, and she was "not breathing well." Fortunately, shots of adrenaline and epinephrine solved the problem.

I was surprised to learn that Rachel had been released

from the hospital a few weeks later without any pre-scribed medication. When I asked how this came about she explained:

> I was acting very well. I was going to therapy. I was
> acting happy. I was telling them that everything was
> fine. . . . I wanted out [of the hospital]. . . . I was
> done. . . . These people had done their best and it
> wasn't working. . . . I wanted my old depressed life
> back.

She went to live with relatives in another state, and, indeed, her depression returned full force. Soon she landed in a state hospital after swallowing fifty-five assorted pills. In contrast to her first stay at a private hospital, Rachel discovered at the public hospital "what people who don't have insurance go through when they're mentally ill." She also found doctors who "weren't fooled quite as easily" by her performances. This time she was put on "liquid Prozac," and "because nothing ever made me mad . . . they purposely put me in a room with someone who had anger problems." This jarring combination, she told me, generated "almost surreal" feelings.

While depression, among women especially, may well result from years of suppressing the self, the emergence of a new, relatively undepressed self can also prove problematic. Rachel described her initial response to Prozac as both remarkable and disquieting:

> Yeah, at first it's wonderful, it's overwhelming; it's
> confusing, it's just such a total change in everything.

It's a change in the way you see things, it's a change
in the way you see yourself. . . . Before that, every day
I woke up I knew what I was going to feel. Once I
started taking that drug, I didn't know. I didn't know
if I was going to wake up happy or if I was going to
wake up sad, [or if] I was going to wake up angry. I
didn't know. For me it made the times I was depressed much harder because if I was depressed all
the time I could deal with it. But if I was happy for a
little while and then I started to get depressed again,
it was tough, it was work, it wasn't as comfortable as
it had been before. And so this made it less normal.
And it made it more uncomfortable. Well, for the first
year I tried real hard to adjust to this new me, to this
new life. I didn't fight the fact that I had to take the
medicine. I knew, after trying to kill myself, obviously, there was something wrong. I needed medication. . . . [But] there's been a persistent confusion
about the real me since I started taking Prozac. The
first drugs I took [the nortriptyline and trazodone]
. . . altered the way I felt, they didn't alter me. They
didn't alter my identity or how I felt about [myself].
[They] altered how I felt at the moment I was taking
the medication . . . because it made me numb. Now, I
don't know who I am.

As you will see in reading Mike's and Emily's accounts
to follow, questions about authenticity of self do not
dominate drug narratives when the medications fail altogether or succeed completely. In cases like Rachel's—

perhaps the most typical of the interviews I conducted—
questions of identity become important when the medications work partially and inconsistently. Much of Rachel's life since her second hospitalization had involved
experimentation with dosage levels as depression regularly "broke through" the medication. In addition, hers
was a history of noncompliance as she tried to discover
whether she could live her life without medications. As
Kay Redfield Jamison observes in her extraordinary memoir *An Unquiet Mind,* "No pill can help [someone] deal
with the problem of not wanting to take pills."[4]

Patients' noncompliance with doctors' orders is a widespread phenomenon and well analyzed in the medical
and social science literatures.[5] While physicians, wedded
to assumptions of rationality, often attribute noncompliance to poor communication between doctors and
patients, sociologists are much more likely to stress the
symbolic meanings attached to aspects of treatment, including medications. When our conversation turned to
her repeated efforts to stop her medications despite the
relief they were providing, Rachel contrasted psychotropic drugs with medications prescribed for physical ailments: "Swallowing pills to deal with emotional pain is
a completely different thing. It's a much harder pill to
swallow."

The special difficulty of using psychiatric medications
is illustrated by another feature of Rachel's life. She had
the double misfortune of suffering from fibromyalgia
as well as depression. Although some researchers have
linked fibromyalgia with psychiatric problems, Rachel is

convinced that her fibromyalgia is physically based. In an inventive interpretive twist she said: "Having fibromyalgia has helped because one of the things they prescribe for people with fibromyalgia is the SSRIs. . . . So [I'm] not just taking it because I'm depressed." She described telling her coworkers, who knew she had been changing medications, "'I went to see a pharmacologist.' [I didn't say] '*psycho*pharmacologist.'" Laughing, she added, "I just left a few syllables off." Rachel explicitly rejected analogies between physical and emotional illnesses:

> I think a physical process and an emotional process are two completely different entities. And having had many physical things wrong with me . . . having had . . . surgery . . . the way that other people look at it is just completely different than the way they look at emotional difficulties. [With] emotional difficulties I think people look down on you. . . . I had knee surgery because my kneecap was in the wrong spot, and so every time I bent my leg, my kneecap would grind against my femur and it tore away all the cartilage. . . . I could not sit and tell my kneecap, "Don't be in this spot, be over here!" You can't change that, that's a physical thing. You have no control over it. You have some control over your emotions.

Certainly all chronic, severe illnesses affect people's identities profoundly.[6] What seems clear from Rachel's comments (which were echoed by others throughout the interviews) is that psychotropic medications have deeper consequences for one's self than do medications for more clearly physical problems. Aside from the stigma that may be attached to psychiatric conditions, prolonged use of psychotropic drugs causes a patient to wonder whether he or she might be a different person when taking medication. Over the years this confusion had led Rachel to try many times to stop taking her psychotropic medication. Her Siddhartha-like search for self befuddled and angered doctors who could not understand why anyone would tamper with the relative health antidepressants provide. As I tried to convey in describing my own short-lived attempt to give up medication, the impulse to do so expressed a yearning for an authentic and integrated self. I understood Rachel when she made comments like these:

> I shouldn't have to take a pill to be happy. I should be able to be happy without medicine.

> I just wish that I didn't need that pill.

> There's always the hope . . . When you first stop taking the medication, the first few weeks you're okay. . . . You're okay because the medicine is still in your system, and I know that. But it gives you kind of this false hope, like, "Look, I haven't taken my medicine in three days and I'm still happy today." And it gives you false hope that you can stop taking it and you'll be okay without it.

At the time of our interview Rachel was nearly fifteen years into her medication career. I cannot say that she had finally embraced medications warmly. It would be more accurate to conclude that she had recognized their value and, after many unsuccessful attempts to leave them behind, she had surrendered to the idea that they would be a constant in her life. She told me, "Prozac saved my life. I honestly think if I didn't go on it, and I didn't experience normal life, I would have attempted suicide again. I wouldn't be sitting here today talking to you." The evidence now seemed firm enough for her to say, with resignation, "I've tried going completely pill-less and it doesn't work out very well for me." At various times she had weaned herself from a number of drugs, always with identical results: "By the time I got off them I was a mess." When I suggested that the bad feelings might be from drug withdrawal, she agreed. However, she now considered it impossible to sort out the connections between mental illness, medication, and self. Rachel had reached the point where continued experimentation to clarify cause and effect was just too costly, both emotionally and physically. When I asked if she still thought about stopping her medications, she replied:

> I don't think I'll get off. No, I'm committed to them now. After going off the Zoloft and trying to go back on it and finding that it didn't work, I think that scared me. I have a lot of other issues when I start taking new drugs. I've always been sort of chemically sensitive. So now when I find one that works . . . If

> the Remeron [a drug she recently began taking]
> works, I will continue taking it. . . . I've definitely
> formed a relationship with Klonopin and with SSRIs.

While Rachel may now be married to medication, it is not
the relationship she wanted. Neither is it an especially stable one:

> I think I'm very, very back and forth. I go through pe-
> riods where I am very resigned to the fact that I will
> be taking these drugs for the rest of my life. Then I
> will go through these short periods where I get mad
> about it. I get upset about it. I say, "Everybody else
> doesn't have to take this. Why do I?" It [uncertainty]
> reemerges from time to time and those are tough pe-
> riods. . . . When I first started to question whether or
> not I should be taking the Prozac . . . it was a daily
> question. It was an everyday [question] when I sat
> and looked at those pills. "Do I take them? Do I not
> take them?" Now, it's maybe a semi-yearly question.

Rachel was between a rock and a hard place. Like many
others, she had become dependent on medications whose
effectiveness is uncertain but whose side effects are often
certainly bad. After so many years, she had lost sight of
the person she might be without medications, and she
had surrendered to a life bounded by them. Her newest
medication, Remeron, captured her dilemma. The drug
knocked her out at night, ensuring sleep, but caused her
"to walk into many more walls than I used to" each morn-

ing. Of course, all of life requires hard choices. All commitments—to people, places, occupations, ideas—are tested constantly as we imagine possibly better alternatives. In addition, all commitments require continuing assessments of who we were, who we have become, and who we might someday be.

Hope and Disillusionment

Mike is an energetic, physically fit man who in his twenties sparred regularly with a regional welterweight champion. I was eager to interview Mike, whose work as a depression support group facilitator I had long admired. Mike often described himself in group meetings as "treatment resistant," so I was especially interested in documenting his thoughts on drugs and illness.[7] When I thanked him for putting aside an evening to talk to me, he explained that mornings were not an option for him, since he suffered from "poverty of thought" until well into the afternoon: "You'd think [in the morning] that I never read anything [and] hadn't been on the planet for the last fifty years, because there's just nothing that can be retrieved. It's horrible."

Although he described the adolescent rebellion of his teenage years as including all-weekend partying, heavy drinking, and a relationship with his father characterized by "pushing each other's buttons," he did well in his small-town prep school, and was even elected class president. As a high school student, he could not have recognized that having "more energy than I knew what to do with and [getting] really wound up at times" were symptoms of mild hypomania (a stage of mania during which individuals entertain grand ideas, are filled with energy, can get along without much sleep, feel extremely creative, and can accomplish an enormous amount of work—a stage that often precedes an episode of psychotic mania). In fact, he was not diagnosed with bipolar illness until his early thirties. Even without a diagnosis, though, he knew by the time he entered college that something was wrong. As a freshman premed major he "got hit with depression and . . . could go to the library for six hours and nothing would sink in." "I did that for a semester," he told me, "and was really messed up and just withdrawn." He did have a capacity for cramming—later seen as connected to hypomania—that sometimes kept him awake for long periods. Indeed, he discovered that "if you stay up long enough the depression will lift. . . . You can go from suicidal, to twenty-four hours without sleep, to being very social, outgoing, and optimistic about life."

Like so many who go for years suffering from an undiagnosed illness, Mike medicated himself. In his case it was with "grass every night before I went to bed," hashish, alcohol, and occasionally amphetamines. The "edge of craziness" he experienced during those years made it impossible to relax without recreational drugs or strenuous physical activity. His taste for danger as a way of combating anxiety led him to downhill skiing "because of the intensity of the speed" and to boxing with the welterweight, who "beat me up four times a week." None of these activities dulled his emotional pain, and he soon left school for a job as a long-distance trucker. The job provided some relief: "When I was out of town and on the road . . . I didn't have anybody telling me what to do." Mike eventually returned to school, went through an "ugly divorce," and entered Alcoholics Anonymous in the belief that his problems were the result of alcohol abuse. Although he stopped drinking, his depression and anxiety persisted, and at age thirty-four, Mike had to face the possibility that there was something deeply wrong with *him*.

While he initially resisted seeing a psychiatrist because he "felt it was humiliating" and "didn't want anybody telling me there was anything wrong with my head," the depression and the desperation it created eventually pushed him into a doctor's office. When I asked Mike if he was also initially resistant to medications, he replied:

> No, I was in so much pain that I really didn't care what I had to take to get out of the pain. When the depression got really bad, I knew that I was drinking to deal with the depression, and I knew that drinking relieved the depression. So . . . I was tuned into the fact that you could do something chemically and relieve the depression. So . . . for me there wasn't any resistance at all.

It is one of the ironies of Mike's long history with medications that only the very first drug he took gave him sustained relief. At that time the drugs most commonly prescribed for depression belonged to a class known as tricyclic antidepressants, one of the earliest of which was amitriptyline: "[My doctor] gave me amitriptyline, which is . . . supposed to take two . . . to six weeks to work. It took two weeks. I felt like a brand-new person. . . . I was amazed."[8] No doubt Mike's later disappointments with a wide array of drugs were deepened by their contrast with this early success. Buoyed by good health and the discovery that he had a natural talent for carpentry, he enthusiastically made plans for a new career. However, "Just about a year to the day, the stuff stopped working." At that point the depression was only momentarily relieved by periods of hypomania:

> Then I started into this pattern of two and a half to three weeks of . . . mild hypomania where I felt really good and was focused and could function. Then I would start going downhill. . . . I was exercising again through all of this. . . . When I started going downhill, I would start intensifying the amount of exercise I did, thinking that . . . I was going back to that runner's high . . . I used to be able to get. But no matter what I did . . . if the depression started on a Sunday, no matter how hard I tried, by Wednesday I would be lying on the bed, curled up and aching . . . in a state of absolute despair and physically aching. And . . . I was saying to myself, "Depression can't make you ache because it's just in my mind. I'm depressed in my head, so how can I be aching from this?" I would be at the point where I would be so depressed I'd just give up. And then I wouldn't even try and help myself. . . . I'd reached the point where [I was] lying in

bed on . . . Wednesday . . . Thursday, possibly Friday, and then, without any effort, I would just come right up out of the depression. And I didn't realize that I was mildly hypomanic at the time.

When, years previously, Mike had returned to an undergraduate program following his truck-driving stint, he had majored in psychology. I asked what he felt about biological and psychological explanations for mental illness. Recalling his success with amitriptyline, he replied with some animation:

I just get really . . . pissed off about all the psychological theories that I've read. . . . When I went back to [college] . . . I was able to go through those [psychological] theories . . . from all different angles to try and understand just what was causing [my] level of depression. Then, after two weeks [on amitriptyline], I said, "Oh man, this [psychology stuff] is just . . . bullshit."

Despite the eventual failure of the medication, Mike's taste of drug success solidified his commitment to a biomedical view of his illness. His experience was profound enough to foster his belief in what the sociologist Allan Horwitz has called "diagnostic psychiatry," with its unflinching commitment to biochemical solutions. Such a belief system is nearly always the backdrop for years of experimentation with a series of medications.[9]

It is hard to overstate the difficulty of starting a new

drug, staying on it for enough time to determine its effects, adjusting doses to minimize side effects, and then weaning yourself off when it doesn't work. In the 1970s Mike quickly worked his way through a series of tricyclics, including nortriptyline, imipramine, and desipramine. He also tried lithium, a natural salt, which was "a major negative event. . . . It just knocked me on my ass." At some point during this period Mike also tried, without success, another category of antidepressants called MAOIs (monoamine oxidase inhibitors), which can cause dangerous reactions, even death, if mixed with certain foods.[10]

Since Mike's doctor believed in giving each medication at least a six-week trial before discarding it, you can imagine how long Mike spent on this exhausting drug merry-go-round. He did the math for me: "If we went through five drugs that didn't work, that could be thirty or forty weeks of drug trials and nothing is working. But when we left them behind we left them behind. . . . If we revisited them it was only in desperation." Then, with the arrival of the SSRIs in the early 1980s, he began another round of experiments, one drug at a time:

> I started going around in a circle again. . . . The SSRIs had come in. Well, the SSRIs were a complete waste. One after another made me sick. Prozac when it first came out was the miracle drug, so . . . I was willing to put up with feeling like nauseated to the point of just about throwing up for about two weeks and staying sick in bed trying to adjust to the Prozac. [I was]

thinking, "Well, what's the alternative? Nothing's working. And this is the drug that's taking people off the back wards." So, you know, it's a reason to hang in there with this. That's how Prozac affected me. . . . Finally after two weeks I stopped taking it. Then I think . . . I started working my way through the SSRIs . . . and they're not working, one after another. Then I get into Paxil. Paxil has me nauseated. . . . I stayed on it for a while . . . trying to adjust to it because of what it did. The first eight hours after I take a Paxil I am sick, really sick. The second eight hours . . . I'm sick and shaky. . . . Then after eight hours of being sick and shaky I start getting a little bit of relief. . . . So I figure, "Okay, maybe I'm going to adjust to this." So I tried this for, you know, a few weeks, but . . . sick and shaky for eight hours is a long time, especially if you don't see any change.

Later Mike talked about the downward spiral created when an illness characterized by feelings of hopelessness does not respond to doctors' best efforts:

I think being knocked down repeatedly, repeatedly disappointed, [is awful]. As I said to a friend of mine, "Just the impact of this illness on your life, the situations it creates, careerwise, financially, socially, relationships, your inability to see a future . . . If you put a normal person that wasn't sick in that situation, it wouldn't be very long before they were seriously depressed." . . . And if you can't get out of it because the

> medication doesn't work . . . I think you get to the
> point where the pain just far outweighs any pleasure
> or satisfaction. . . . When you get to the point where
> the illness has you in agony day after day all day long,
> you want to take yourself out. You're only sticking
> around because of the guilt trip . . . thinking . . . what
> impact it would have on people you love.

Like others who stumble from one drug to another, Mike became an expert on medications, often feeling that he knew more than the doctors who were treating him, particularly about his own drug regimens. I have often heard variants on Mike's observation, "When you're listening to a professional talk, they don't really get it at the depth of someone that's lived it." In my experience patients are grateful when doctors admit the incompleteness of their knowledge and the truth that their recommendation of a particular drug is largely guesswork. Mike especially admired the doctor who "when he gave me the medication . . . the first time . . . was truthful. . . . He said, 'We're playing black box medicine here. We don't really know what we're doing.'"

To illustrate how patients must sometimes take drug matters into their own hands because of doctors' lack of comprehension, Mike detailed what he had to do to discontinue Klonopin, a highly habituating medication in a family of drugs called benzodiazepines, which also includes Ativan, Xanax and Valium.[11] He began to realize that the Klonopin, which he had been taking for anxiety, ultimately had a boomerang effect: "The first Klonopin of the day would have a good effect for about two and a half . . . hours. [However], the depression and anxiety would come back more intense, and then the next [pill] wasn't effective." He added:

> Since I had smoked and drank . . . I said [to myself], "It's bad enough to be addicted to stuff that you can go down to the corner store and get immediately if you wanted to. It's another thing to be addicted to something that you have to call up somebody [to get]." So I decided to come off the Klonopin, but I didn't tell the doctor I was going to come off it.

Mike had learned through painful experience that a drug with a very short "half-life" (the amount of time it takes for the blood level of a drug to drop by 50 percent) can shortly make you feel that you have far less than half a life.[12]

Like Mike, I often worry about whether, after fifteen years of use, I am addicted to Klonopin. Therefore, I listened intently when Mike explained that the only way he could stop taking Klonopin was to lie to his doctor. Believing that doctors often grossly underestimate the difficulty of giving up such drugs, Mike "didn't want them deciding how fast I should be able to come off it." He tapered off the medication over several months while "I just kept getting the prescriptions. . . . I'd [even] keep track of when it was time to fill the next one and even if I had a hundred tablets left I still filled the next one." When, finally, he was no longer taking the Klonopin, he told the doctor that he wanted to stop, and, as expected, he was given a plan that would have required tapering off in three weeks. Mike expressed disbelief that doctors could be unaware of the difficulty of discontinuing an addictive drug:

> Yeah, I'm just amazed, I'm amazed. . . . Why hasn't this been figured out? Because people know about the other benzodiazepines. . . . I know someone that went through Valium withdrawal and also went through alcohol withdrawal. And he said alcohol withdrawal, which can kill you, was a piece of cake compared to getting off Valium. It took something like two and a half years and he was still reacting to it. . . . I think that the cure was worse than the illness. I think that the Klonopin . . . if it was doing something for me in the beginning, was no longer working as effectively. And it was actually making me worse with that boomerang effect. Plus, what I did notice when I got off the Klonopin is [that] my memory improved dramatically and I seemed to have less apathy, less lethargy. When I heard other people like really suffering, going through the withdrawal, and sometimes they would actually even have to go to the hospital, I was really quite pleased with myself that I had handled it that way. With all my stupidity caused by the depression and cognitive distortion and chaos, at least I thought to myself, "Well, you did yourself a favor there."

Among the few drugs in recent years that have dulled Mike's depression is an atypical antidepressant called Wellbutrin.[13] On Wellbutrin he "felt sort of like going out and dancing and drinking and whatever else came to mind." However, as Mike found out the hard way, Wellbutrin has been known to cause mania in some people. Mike had been doing well on Wellbutrin until he reached a dose of 300 milligrams while on a trip to a neighboring state. At that point "something kicked in." He described the encroaching mania: "I felt like I was going to go through the roof. . . . [It was] almost too intense. It's almost like I wanted to escape it." Appropriately, Mike decreased the amount of Wellbutrin he was taking, but he never told his doctor what had happened when he was away. He believed that psychiatrists "are afraid of mania. They're afraid of mania and I was taking the medication that pushed me into mania or something that was very close to it. . . . So, knowing that doctors get absolutely paranoid about mania, [I said nothing]. Some doctors won't even give bipolars antidepressants. They'd rather see them go through their life depressed . . . which I think is criminal." Mike continued to experiment with dosage levels, but questions of noncompliance eventually became moot when, a few months later, the salutary effects of the Wellbutrin disappeared.

While Mike was grateful for whatever small relief he sometimes got from the "next" drug, even the best ones "still leave me in hell." He questioned the pharmaceutical companies' assertions that their drugs "work" for 80 percent of people suffering from depression.[14] Does this include the people who experience only incremental relief, or those who trade one set of symptoms for another? The claim is misleading, Mike contended, because "people think of working as some significant and meaningful relief from pain." When I suggested that drugs sometimes only move people from the eighth to the seventh of Dante's circles of hell, Mike laughed and said, "Right. . . . You're standing on your head in the mud instead of having your toes burned. . . . It's just . . . very deceptive advertising and it's unethical."

Given his history, it is testimony to Mike's spirit and courage that he still searched for solutions. Although he continued to hope for new medications that might pierce even *his* mood disorder, at the time of our talk he was focusing on alternative treatments, particularly supplements. He used fish oil, flaxseed oil, Sami, St. John's Wort, and kava kava, among other things. We laughed about the latest remedy he was considering—pig vitamins. Six months before our interview he had heard a grain and feed salesman talk about "a certain mix of vitamins . . . and minerals that [farmers] give to aggressive pigs. . . . Everyone's joking that . . . we're going to listen to a salesman and a pig farmer . . . and that's going to turn our life around." Apparently, though, some unorthodox doctors had taken the pig vitamins seriously, and reports on the Internet claimed astounding success. Mike was looking into the matter.

Toward the end of the interview I asked Mike the two questions I routinely asked all my interviewees: "What is the most difficult thing about using psychiatric drugs?" and "What would you most want those who read my book to know about psychiatric drug use?" Here's how Mike responded to the first question:

> I think the first thing that came to mind as the most difficult thing about taking them is the fact that they don't work [for me]. I don't think that if they worked I'd have any problems taking them. If I was feeling very well I might be even more worried about what they were going to do to my wonderful life [in terms of health] down the road. But I don't get down the road too far with them now, you know.

And about the message he wanted to convey to readers:

> I would like to have it just spelled out in plain language . . . the fact that one-third of the people respond well [to medications] and the rest don't respond well. The fact [is] that one-third don't respond at all. . . . Just get the truth out there and get it out just . . . point-blank.

Because of the difficulties in determining whether treatments "work," no one really knows the true effectiveness of either talk or drug therapies. There is no way to affirm or disprove the validity of Mike's last claim that a third of those with affective disorders are treatment resistant. What does seem clear is that responses to medications exist along a continuum from cure to failure. While we cannot know just how those who suffer from depression, anxiety, and bipolar illness are statistically arranged along this continuum, there seems little doubt that medications do not routinely cure mood disorders. At the same time, as Emily's account will show, medications are sometimes absolute life savers.

Fear Strikes Out

One of my intellectual heroes is a writer named Ernest Becker, who in the 1970s won a Pulitzer Prize for his book *The Denial of Death.*[15] The provocative theme of this book, pushed along by a psychoanalytic imagination, is that the meaning of life is contingent on the knowledge that we will someday die. Much of our creativity in work and other spheres of life, Becker argues, is motivated by efforts to deny our own mortality. Yet the reality of our eventual demise continually pushes in on us: "The knowledge of death is reflective and conceptual, and [lower] animals are spared it. . . . But to live a whole lifetime with the fate of death haunting one's dreams and even the most sun-filled days—that's something else."[16] Emily, at age fifty, was terrified of dying and had twice experienced serious medical problems followed by life-threatening depressions.

Early in my interviews I asked people a number of demographic questions, including their religion. Although she had been raised Catholic and attended parochial schools prior to high school, Emily had "stopped going to church as soon as I was on my own." Later she had two children, both of whom were baptized and received communion even while she was saying to herself, "Why am I doing this? I'm a hypocrite." Soon thereafter, Emily fell away from the Church completely despite feeling that "part of me really believes in spirituality." Emily was still searching for a source of spiritual comfort, and this, she explained, was "part of the problem." When I asked her to elaborate she said:

> I am so afraid of dying. . . . I look forward to a lot of important things to do in my life, and so to me death is so final. It's the scariest thing in the world. I don't want to think about it. . . . I have no control over it so it bothers me. And part of it is because I don't believe in an afterlife. I don't have these things like God [to] get me through this. I don't feel like there's anything out there that's going to get me through all this.

Although Emily's anxiety disorder and depression had not been diagnosed until after her medical emergencies, her life-distorting anxiety was probably rooted in her childhood.[17] Her father was "very blue collar" and a "very bad alcoholic" who drifted from job to job, causing the family to constantly totter at the brink of poverty. Emily's mother, who never wanted to work, "was in a constant state of anger, always yelling at us [Emily and two brothers] because she was frustrated and angry with him." When Emily was eleven or twelve, nights were filled with parental fights and her father's repeated declaration, "As soon as these kids get old I'm leaving you." "That used to scare me," she said. "I had no control. . . . We used to do everything to make my father happy, but it never worked." Given these circumstances, it makes sense that Emily remembered "always being afraid of things and getting very anxious feelings. . . . My stomach got the fight-or-flight syndrome all the time. [I was] feeling insecure, unsafe."

During her college years Emily may have lacked a spiritual life, but she certainly had an independent spirit. She had little anxiety about resisting family expectations: "I wasn't the type of girl that was [too] anxious . . . to do things. I used to do things I knew would get me in trouble, but I still did them." Imagine the taboos violated in a white, working-class family during the 1960s when Emily fell in love with a black man. After seven years social convention eventually destroyed the relationship:

> He was a black person and my family just absolutely couldn't stand it. He broke up with me because he couldn't take it anymore. And that was my first real bout with depression. I remember losing like fifteen pounds, being very sad. It was a loss, right. But I was able to pick myself up . . . and get going. . . . I could still function. I went to work. No one knew I was even suffering. I was really good at dealing with it.

In many ways Emily's biography testifies to how completely anxiety can be compartmentalized. The things that terrify one person cause no difficulty for another. In her job as an educational administrator, for example, Emily had no difficulty making public presentations, the most common social phobia by far. Although she had experienced low levels of anxiety during most of her adult life, Emily was never hobbled by it and always navigated gracefully through some of life's toughest challenges, including a divorce. Whatever difficulties she suffered were largely invisible to those around her. That all changed, however, when she experienced a series of life-threatening complications following a hysterectomy. Unable to "go on hormone replacement therapy as a result of the anesthesia and the hospital not paying attention, I developed multiple pulmonary embolisms. I came home [and] didn't know what happened. I was in excruciating pain." As a result:

> I went back to the hospital [and] they told me that if I had stayed [at home] another day I would have died. I was close to death and I was . . . in intensive care for three days. So finally I was getting better, and the more I was in the hospital, the more scared I became, every day. And I hated being there, but for some reason I started feeling really scared about my life, like I was going to die or something bad was going to happen to me again. As I was getting better, you would think I would start feeling better, but I started feeling worse. . . . The doctors were telling me I was getting better. Everybody was saying, "Are you ready to go home?" And when I came home . . . that night I could not sleep at all and I had the shakes. So I thought, "Oh, I'm having drug withdrawal" because when I was in the hospital I was on tons of drugs for pain-

killing and all that. So I shook all night long and I woke up the next morning still shaking. I couldn't eat. My stomach had that horrible feeling. I was crying and that was the beginning of my depression. . . . It was very bad. I wasn't eating at all. I was down to like 103 pounds. I was out of work. I couldn't go to work. I couldn't get out of bed. . . . It was really bad and everybody said to me, "You have to go see someone."

Depression's pain is significantly multiplied when it is disbelieved by others. Emily first dragged herself out of bed to see an internist, who insisted there was nothing wrong with her and repeatedly asked, "Why are you doing this?" Similarly, Emily's mother expressed the familiar pull-yourself-up-by-your-bootstraps mentality:

After this experience my mother and I haven't been as close because I could hear her saying, "I'm going to go upstairs and make her get out of bed and she's going to eat this tonight if I have to throw it down her face." You know, she was so unsympathetic, and it really, really hurt me and made me mad. And I remember saying to her, "Do you think I'd be doing this if I could snap out of it?"

Naming Emily's illness as depression was difficult because most people associate depression with mental pain only. In her case, "the physical pain was worse than the labor pain when I had two children. It was horrible. . . .

I could not [keep] food [down]. I would throw u
started eating. . . . It was that fight-or-flight syndrome.
Oddly, it was a neighbor who suggested that her symptoms might indicate depression. Looking back, Emily
found it ironic that her depression had been triggered by
a fear of dying:

> Nothing interested me. All I would do is just lie there.
> I remember thinking, "You know, if I died right now
> I'd be fine." . . . What's so funny about it is that I was
> so afraid of dying, but when I was in my depression I
> was sitting there thinking, "You know, it's okay if I
> die. It might be better than this." Because the way I
> felt was so crappy. I never thought of killing myself, I
> can honestly say that, [but] I remember thinking, "If
> somebody else killed me it would have been fine."
> Like if somebody broke into the house and stabbed
> me to death that would have been okay [laughs].

The power of antidepressant medications seems most
incontrovertible when relief occurs precisely on the time
schedule predicted and is experienced as a complete cure.
Emily finally found her way to a psychiatric nurse, who
prescribed Klonopin and Prozac and told her: "Klonopin
will really help you now because the Prozac won't kick
in for about six weeks." In response, Emily exclaimed, "I
can't wait six weeks. I'm going to die before six weeks!"
However, the Klonopin, taken three or four times a day,
dulled her pain, and within two weeks things began to
change:

> About four and a half, almost five weeks . . . it started
> being good. And then by six weeks it was like . . . I
> was feeling no pain. I was eating, back to work, con-
> centrating, wanting to go out, get on with my life, ev-
> erything was great. Everything was great. And how
> can it not be the drug? When they tell you you'll feel
> better in five to six weeks, is it your mind making you
> feel better because they told you [you would im-
> prove], or is it the drug? I truly believe it's the drug. I
> really do.

Having good friends at work who were anxiously following her situation allowed Emily to be forthright about
medications once she returned to her office: "I started
telling people myself, 'I'm on Prozac [and it's] saving
me.'" A lapsed Catholic had experienced a miracle.

Even miracles can tarnish over time. As 50 to 60 percent of people using SSRIs discover, the drugs can significantly affect libido. Emily's enthusiasm for Prozac was
at least slightly diminished when she realized that "it affected my sex life somewhat. Not that I didn't want sex—
that's not the problem—but I had a very hard time having
an orgasm, and [the nurse] said that's one of the side effects of the medication." The matter of sexual side effects
points to one of the central themes of this book: drug-
taking is a social event that extends well beyond the pill
and the person taking it. Our views about medications
are clearly shaped by people close to us.

Emily's boyfriend, Richard, began to say, "You're doing

great. Why don't you see if you can go off. . . . You had a hysterectomy. Your hormones were out of whack. You're not depressed. You're a happy person. Maybe now that you're past that you'll be fine." It was hard for Emily to dismiss such observations in the context of her evolving relationship with Richard. She told me: "I felt like Richard was working so hard to please me, and I started feeling guilty, and then I was thinking, 'Well, he's going to get disinterested in me, and then what am I going to do?' It did become something I thought of." So, despite the advice of her nurse practitioner, Emily went off the Prozac. She found that "my sex life was back to normal [and] everything was great." Indeed, everything remained fine for nearly three years, until an annual medical checkup revealed a low white blood cell count. Although tests showed no signs of cancer and the doctor explained that she might be someone with a normally low count, Emily began to worry: "I'm a walking time bomb to get cancer. Cancer's around the corner. I don't have it now but it's coming. It's coming." Within days she fell into a "major depression just like the last time."

Finding her way out of depression's tangle proved more difficult the second time. Emily explained that her torment was extended by an arrogant psychiatrist who claimed to know what was best for her. Despite her prior success with Prozac, the new doctor insisted that another drug, BuSpar, was unquestionably the right choice for her. Although the BuSpar did make her feel better after four or five days, it then abruptly stopped working. When

Emily reported her experience the doctor remained convinced that BuSpar would work if she gave it more time. While the pain of anxiety and depression felt essentially the same as during her first episode, this time she told herself, "I have to go back to work":

> I got myself out of bed and went to work because I
> was afraid to be home alone. I don't know why, but
> this time was a little different. So I'd go in to work
> and close my door. I don't know what good that did.
> I got out of the house but I'd close the door. I
> couldn't do a damn thing.

Emily's agony fostered a growing dissatisfaction with her doctor:

> I went to him out of desperation one last time. And I
> said, "BuSpar is not working." I said, "Why aren't you
> putting me on another antidepressant?" I think we
> wasted four weeks. I could have been on another anti-
> depressant for four weeks and I wasn't. I said, "I can't
> take this anymore." He said, "Okay, I'll put you on
> Effexor." He said Effexor works a little faster. And [he
> also prescribed] some other drug. I don't even re-
> member what the other was. Now I'm getting really
> nervous. I'm saying, "This guy doesn't know what the
> hell he's doing." I thought he was experimenting
> with me. And he thought he knew everything. He
> wasn't listening to me when I told him Prozac
> worked. He kept telling me, "No, you don't need

Prozac." And blah, blah, blah. And Richard said,
"We're not going to him anymore."

With the help of colleagues at work, Emily found her way to a new psychiatrist, let's call her Dr. Hernandez, whom she came to love. When I asked what made the new doctor so good, Emily replied:

> Her gentle mannerism, her voice. . . . When I started seeing her she would call me at home to see how I was doing. And whenever I called her—no matter where she was—I got a phone call back within ten minutes. I thought she really cared about me and wanted to see me get better. And she made me feel that taking the medications [she prescribed] was the right thing to do.

Emily's comments confirm the obvious point that patients want doctors who listen well and genuinely care about them. Perhaps less obvious is the real possibility, contrary to the purely biological view of medicine, that the effectiveness of medications is intimately linked to patients' faith and trust in those who prescribe them.

Emily's earliest encounters with her new doctor reveal another important dimension of psychiatric drug use: Patients ascribe very different meanings to different medications. They carry around in their heads a kind of hierarchy of medications based on their relative acceptability. When Dr. Hernandez suggested that she try an SSRI called Celexa because it presumably had fewer side effects than Prozac, Emily was happy to comply:

> And then an interesting thing happened. [Dr. Hernandez] said, "I want you to take some Ritalin." So I said, "Well, why am I going to take Ritalin?" She said, "Until the Celexa kicks in the Ritalin will give you an energy boost. It will get you out of bed and get you going." I said, "I don't want to take Ritalin" because I always thought Ritalin was a *real* drug, a drug addict's drug. It's an amphetamine or something? People take it like speed. I thought this drug would make me feel real good, like high. . . . So it scared me.

After several days of wrangling, the combination of Dr. Hernandez's calm demeanor and her own continuing panic finally persuaded Emily to try the medication, with the happy result that "I started feeling pretty good. I said, 'Wow, there's something to this.'"

Within a few weeks the miracle of medication repeated itself and Emily felt "absolutely fantastic." At the time of our conversation she had been taking a combination of Celexa and Wellbutrin. The Wellbutrin had been added because Celexa had produced the same sexual side effects she had experienced with Prozac. While that problem has been solved, the medications did blunt her feelings somewhat: "I am able to feel anger and I'm able to cry, but I do notice that I feel a little more apathetic than I want to be." However, compared with her awful depressions, the drug's side effects seem modest. Once Emily began to improve, Dr. Hernandez told her that "if you have had two bouts of what I had . . . you need to be on the medication for the rest of your life." The doctor then asked, "How do you feel about that?" Emily was quick to reply:

> I'm absolutely staying on it for the rest of my life. I don't want to ever go through this again. [I] wake up in the morning feeling fine. I feel like I'm back to my old self. . . . I don't feel like I have extremes anymore. I'm just more even. I went for a colonoscopy last week because when you turn fifty you should. And I wasn't even worried about it. So I thought that was good. I could have been anxious, feeling worried about that. That's not to say that I won't be anxious again if something bad happens. I probably will, but I think the medications will help me not go into the real depression.

Toward the end of our meeting my conversation with Emily took an unexpected and interesting turn. For more than two hours her story had seemed to be one of complete conversion to psychiatric medicines; I was convinced that after her wonderful responses to drugs, Emily felt that medication was the only alternative. While there turned out to be relatively few fissures in her belief that depression is a biomedical disorder, they did exist. When I asked her if she wanted to elaborate on anything we had talked about, Emily acknowledged that there was something that bothered her about drugs: "People who are really spiritual, I bet they're not the people you are interviewing [who are] on these drugs." Our conversation came full circle when Emily once again expressed a longing for a spiritual life, which she thought might insulate her from anxiety and depression even more effectively than Celexa and Wellbutrin:

> Part of me thinks that maybe if I was more spiritual, I could deal with this stuff better and I wouldn't need the drugs. . . . I guess I'd like to hear people who are spiritual say, "Well, I took the drugs but now I don't need them anymore because I've found more spirituality [and] that helped me through it. . . . See, there's this big part of me that thinks, "It's the medication that's making me feel better." [However, I also think that] "if I was spiritual would I still need it?" I don't know. I watch a news program where somebody lost a child, and they're not even crying. They're so composed, and they're saying, "The Lord, you know, is praying for me." They bring up the Lord and their spirituality. . . . If one of my kids got killed, I'm afraid of what I would do. I'm not even sure if the Celexa would help me. And these people are so composed, and they're dealing with it, and I go, "Wow, is that what spirituality does for you?" It's better than a drug! If that works for these people, then maybe I should be doing that instead of the drugs, you know? But I don't know how to make myself feel that way. I just marvel that [spirituality] does for them what the drug does for me.

Emily's words suggest a line of thinking that I have often heard from depressed people over the years.[18] During the research for my earlier book on depression, I was struck by the number of people I interviewed who had found great comfort from a variety of spiritual forms, especially Eastern religious and meditative practices. Perhaps there are, as Emily supposed, people whose spirituality frees them from the need for pills. However, most of those with whom I have spoken saw medicine and spirituality as acting jointly. Spiritually inclined people with depression seem to have embraced, far more than others, the Buddhist notion that life's pain is normal. Consequently, many of them have replaced expectations of "cure" with the more spiritual goal of "transformation." Spirituality, with its emphasis on personal transformation, cannot cure depression but certainly helps some people manage it with equanimity and grace.

Emily's longing for a deeper spiritual life and a more holistic approach to her suffering suggests a still deeper truth about illness, medicine, and humanity. As Emily's experience with Dr. Hernandez suggests, people feel better when their doctors see them as whole persons rather than as just a bundle of symptoms. Conventional medicine too often ignores that real healing is a matter of both body and spirit. Indeed, the most humane and effective healing requires treating both cells and souls.

Chapter 3

Married to Medication

It was like I'm going to be on the medication every day for the rest of my life. It was a realization. . . . This is it, and I kind of just tried to accept that. It took me a while to finally get used to that. . . . Eventually the medication just became habit. I wouldn't have to think about it . . . I mean, you brush your teeth so that you don't get cavities, but you just do it because it's habit. So that's what I think I eventually got to. And the pills stopped representing the mental illness to me.

—female psychology student,
aged 21

I once received a fortune cookie that captured the central thesis of this chapter. The fortune read: "An unexpected relationship will become permanent." The fifty people I interviewed for this project could not have known they were making a lifelong commitment to a medical view of their depression when out of desperation they chose to begin taking psychotropic drugs. They had laid the cornerstone for a life circumscribed by pills. Most are married to medications.

After thirty-seven years of marriage, I cannot imagine my life as a single person. Like all long-term relationships, marriage is characterized by rituals that over time become so routine we take them for granted. For example, my wife always gets home from work by 6:15 P.M. If she were to arrive much later I would begin to worry. Everything from eating dinner to getting ready for bed to coupon clipping is relatively predictable. After so long together daily life carries few big surprises. Ours, like most long-term marriages, has also passed through distinct phases (for instance, becoming acclimated to marriage, having children, balancing work and family, dealing with teenagers, sending children out into the world, becoming grandparents). Although all relationships have their bumpy moments, love and a shared history give us great confidence that our partnership will last.

Any analogy, taken too far, strains credibility and potentially undermines analysis. In this chapter I mean for the "married to medication" imagery to be a device for thinking about questions of commitment, what Herbert Blumer has called a "sensitizing concept."[1] Of course, relationships with humans and relationships with drugs are very different: while psychiatrists may talk about "listening" to drugs like Prozac (that is, carefully observing their effects) in order to establish diagnoses, such interactions hardly approximate human conversations. Still, human beings do react to drugs, and our relationships with them unquestionably influence the way we lead our lives. The analogy also holds in that, as with marriages, some relationships with drugs involve love at first sight (or first swallow), some soon end in disillusionment, some are initially rocky and then smooth out over time, some are always conflict-ridden, some involve unhealthy dependencies, some end in divorce after many years, and some become lifelong commitments.

Peter Berger and Hansfried Kellner once wrote a provocative essay entitled "Marriage and the Social Construction of Reality."[2] Their fundamental argument is that marriage may be understood as a process through which two people construct a "joint reality." Two strangers begin a relationship with their independent realities. The possibility of an enduring relationship is partly dependent on whether the two prospective partners have enough in common—values, tastes, attitudes—to foresee making a commitment. The change from being strangers to being intimates involves partners reshaping friendships, interests, and goals in order to move from their independent realities to one jointly held. Similarly, we might say that *any* new commitment, whether to another person, to a career, to a religion, or to medication, involves embracing new realities. In particular, here I am interested in detailing the process through which people begin to embrace a biomedical version of reality. Commitment to taking psychotropic drugs requires acceptance of psychiatry's version of what causes emotional suffering and what should be done to relieve it.

As with the adoption of any belief system, commitment to a medical explanation for emotional distress evolves over time. Most people don't suddenly embrace the notion that they suffer from faulty brain chemistry and need medication to feel better. Typically, they move through a series of life experiences that either strengthen or weaken their newly constructed drug realities. My conversation with Sarah illustrates the process through which someone can go from resistance to taking drugs to the view that "this [drug-taking] is the way I am. This is what I'll need to do for the rest of my life."

Sarah and I had been friends for many years before we sat down to talk about medications. I had known for a long time that her son's schizophrenia dominated her personal life, but I knew relatively little about her own struggles with depression and pill use. Sarah looks much younger than her fifty-six years. She is tall, graceful, and very articulate about her life. I quickly learned that her depression dated from her teenage years and that, like me, she suffered from debilitating insomnia that magnified her misery. Her relationship with drugs had begun with addiction to over-the-counter sleep medications, a secret she had kept from everyone:

> I discovered that Benadryl knocked me out. . . . I was hung over from it the next day, but I slept. They tell you to take two capsules or whatever, and I just needed one to sleep. But eventually I needed two. Eventually two didn't work so I took three. Eventually three didn't work so I took four. . . . And that's when I would go into the drug store and research the ingredient labels . . . so that I could find other stuff that would knock me out but have a different ingredient. And it was a lot of work [laughter], you know,

reading all those ingredient labels. . . . Well, I didn't
go in with a notebook, but I would put my glasses on
and stand there in that . . . aisle for over-the-counter
sleeping medications. . . . And yeah, I would stand
there for a long time. I'm sure their security cameras
were all homing in on this woman who was spending
all this time reading labels. . . . But then the same
thing happened with [another medication] that happened with the Benadryl. I started with a minimal
dose and it worked great. I took the full dose and
then eventually I needed more and [then] I started
mixing them. . . . Nobody knew. Nobody had a clue.

Although Sarah admitted to a certain measure of
shame connected with her secret drug life, she made a
sharp distinction between over-the-counter medications
and prescribed medications. At one point, she told me,
her family doctor had prescribed Valium because she was
a "nervous lady":

I refused to fill it. I didn't want to take prescription
Valium. . . . I knew very well that I was flawed, but . . .
somehow I could fool myself . . . if I weren't taking a
prescription drug. . . . It was something about that
written prescription for a psychiatric drug that . . .
just doomed me for life.

Sarah's history with nonprescription drugs was not
shared by anyone else I interviewed, but her initial resistance to prescribed medications was very common. Also

common was her later shift, out of desperation, to willingness to take antidepressants. When a therapist finally told her that she needed to see a psychiatrist, she responded: "It's such hell; it's so horrible. A couple of months ago I would have refused, but now I know I need to go."

Once having crossed the line into the world of prescribed medications, Sarah nearly instantly fell in love with Prozac. She could sleep and "felt like a new person." Unhappily, she later became so agitated that sitting still was impossible. She realized that Prozac was not the right drug for her. What followed was experimentation with a string of medications, each of which had its flaws. Almost every visit to the doctor involved changing medications: "I got off [each] of them because I would complain that I thought that it was doing this or that and I just didn't want to take it. I wanted something else." Eventually she turned to Ativan, a powerful benzodiazepine, which at the time of our interview she had been taking for many years. "I am addicted," she told me. "I am a drug addict." Just as I have given myself over to Klonopin, Sarah could not contemplate the prospect of stopping Ativan. She believed it helped her sleep and didn't know "what would happen to me if I had to withdraw from Ativan." After two decades of using a variety of psychiatric medications Sarah had come to believe that she couldn't live without her several prescribed drugs: "I'm not well, but I'm better than I would be without them." Like so many others I talked to, Sarah had moved over time from resistance to acceptance:

Now I fully embrace the idea that I have major psychiatric problems and I need the medication. And now I'm glad for the relief it gives me. But it was a long, long road. . . . It took me decades, twenty years or so, to get to the point where I don't mind having the prescriptions. . . . I just wanted to be like everyone else and not [take medications]. I mean, there is still a real stigma . . . attached to psychiatric medications. . . . [But] I just know now that I need it and I'm going to take it and that's it.

Then she added wistfully, "There's still a part of me that wishes I didn't have to take them for the rest of my life."

My own experience, Sarah's, and that of most of the people I interviewed suggest clear regularities in the way distressed people "come around" to taking psychiatric medications. Typically, individuals feel a strong resistance to entering the world of psychiatrists and pills. Eventually they are overcome by feelings of unhappiness and out of desperation agree to try medication. Once having embarked on a search for comfort and well-being through medications, the newly minted patients are persuaded by doctors and family to experiment with drugs until they find the "right one." At a point, most "settle" on a drug regimen which, although far from perfect, is better than their earlier relationships with drugs. Periodically, they make efforts to change things in the hope of increasing their happiness, but after several years the idea of stopping drugs altogether seems impossible. Long-term use of medication leads them to believe that change would be wholly disruptive to their lives, that, all things considered, their lives are better with pills than they would be without them. This process of becoming committed to drugs can be seen as having four stages: desperation, experimentation, engagement, and marriage.

Desperation

These days many young people resist forming permanent relationships until their late twenties or early thirties. However, as the iconic television sitcoms *Sex and the City* and *Friends* convey, eventually constructing an intimate relationship is not so easy for twenty-somethings. It may not be an exaggeration to say that intimacy in America has become a kind of social problem. Having postponed commitments in favor of careers, young men and women wishing to start a family may begin to feel a sense of desperation as they enter their thirties.

Driven by a sense of urgency, young adults may seek help by signing up for expensive dating services, placing personal ads in classified columns, cruising Internet chat rooms, or attending special singles events to meet potential mates. Similarly, many people suffering from depression often "go it alone" for years before seeking professional help as a last resort. Like Sarah, many strongly resist the idea of turning to psychiatrists and psychiatric drugs for their pain. To do so means crossing an identity line from being "troubled" to being "sick."

Over and over I heard people express the same feelings as Jack, a long-term sufferer of manic depression, who recounted his initial reaction to drugs:

> Taking that pill becomes a prominent identity set
> that says one major part of who I am is this ill part of
> me. And it's not the kind of illness that I'm proud of.
> It's the kind of illness that somehow I should
> beat. . . . If I were a well-formed human being, I could
> beat this. That's the stuff that went into my mind.

For most of those I interviewed, nonmedical efforts to deal with their pain eventually failed, and at some point their misery engulfed them. However much they wanted to avoid medicalizing their problem, they believed they had run out of options. Desperation pushed them into doctors' offices and began a radical reconstruction of their reality:

> We started talking about medication and at this
> point I submitted to medication. . . . I finally submit-
> ted. That's the word I used. And I just realized that I
> had to do something because I was desperate. (male
> media consultant, aged 52)

> I was very, very resistant to it [medication]. Some peo-
> ple [I knew] were on medication and I was like, "Oh,
> wow, you really must have bad problems." . . . And
> then I'd listen to them, and I really started . . . feeling
> like, "Oh, I'm not alone." . . . I was [still] really ner-

vous about taking Prozac. I thought [Prozac] was this big huge medicine. I was literally afraid . . . of how it would affect me. I didn't know if I would be the same person. Through therapy I came to realize, "I'm in a lot of pain and I don't know why I'm being a martyr about it." And I decided, I'm going to look into taking medication because I'm tired of this pain. . . . I was way down in the well. (female technical writer, aged 50)

It would be too formulaic to say that people embrace medicines only when desperation overtakes resistance, as though these two forces were inevitable and clearly measurable opposing energies. While some degree of resistance was clearly the norm, several of those I interviewed welcomed without reservation the prospect that pills might ease their pain. For them, beginning a relationship with medication did not seem to raise issues of identity:

I was fighting to get on medication. . . . In high school I was extremely depressed and I reached out for help, and as a sixteen-, seventeen-year-old high school student, it's hard. I'm male [and] it's hard to do that. And I was at the point where I would have just taken anything to make myself feel better. I mean, if they could give me a pill, I would be happy. Sounds good to me. . . . It could be seen as an easy way out, but . . . I didn't know of any other way. (male peace activist, aged 22)

[There was] no resistance. I was absolutely desperate, you know. I spent nine months thinking I was going to be assassinated by the CIA, not sleeping, thinking that my whole office was under surveillance. And I didn't really know I was sick, but I was desperate to do some sleeping. (female entrepreneur, aged 52)

Thus far, I have been describing the path toward medication as an emotionally complicated and difficult *choice* made in the face of desperation. Although people may feel coerced into a relationship with drugs by the severity of their symptoms, they have, in the end, still made a choice. The situation is different when mental illness appears in its most vicious forms: in such cases a sufferer's relationship with medication may begin, literally, as an instance of "involuntary commitment":

I was in the hospital for a long time. I was in the hospital for a total of seven months over two different years. . . . The first time, in 1971, they . . . didn't call me manic-depressive. They didn't know about manic depression. . . . So the first year, when I was hospitalized for four months, I don't even know what they wrote. I mean, did they write down "schizophrenic"? They certainly didn't tell me that. Did they write down "borderline"? They didn't tell me that. They didn't know what to do with me. They wanted to just calm me down. And so they gave me Thorazine and Haldol and Stelazine, and you know, whatever they

could. . . . Just calm me down. (female office worker,
aged 60)

I had no understanding of what was happening to
me at all. On the day of this manic experience, I was
taken by the police to the emergency room. And because they didn't know what was happening, they
then put me in a padded cell. And that gave me the
greatest fright of anything I'd ever experienced. And
then I was taken from the padded cell to go and sleep
in the psych ward. And the next morning I was taken
to see a psychiatrist. I hadn't had a shower. . . . I
didn't feel human. . . . That was when I started on
lithium. With no explanation of what lithium was or
did. (female writer, aged 58)

Whatever the particular route that leads people to
medication, when drugs are first prescribed for them,
they rarely foresee a permanent relationship. At this early
point in their illness career, they may view their connection with medication as a kind of chance encounter, an
association that will help them get past a difficult time in
their lives. Few envision a tie that will bind them to doctors, pills, and other therapies for years to come:

I felt there was something wrong. I think I knew
there was something wrong. I don't think I knew that
it would be with me for the rest of my life. I thought
there was some kind of hope for change. And that it
was sort of a phase, even when I thought something

was wrong with me for going through this phase. (female graduate student, aged 29)

Most people tread slowly and gingerly as they take their first steps into a new world of pills and medical explanations for their emotional problems. The desperation born of intolerable pain may have melted resistance to antidepressants, but initiates into an alien psychiatric culture are justified in questioning the legitimacy of their diagnoses:

One psychiatrist told me in a passageway in the hospital, not even in an office or anything. But he said, "You have a serious mental illness, and it will make a predictable life almost impossible for you." It was one heck of a message. So it was better to deny such a message than to take that seriously. Because unless you can say, "This man is off his hit," then you might as well crawl into a hole. So there were good reasons for denying it. (female writer, aged 58)

The diagnosis was wrong of me. [I thought,] "You [doctor] don't really know what I am because you don't really know who I am." So I felt that no one really saw who I was and no one could tell me who I was. (female sociology student, aged 20)

As Howard Becker describes it, commitments are rarely made consciously and definitively at a given moment in time.[3] Rather, they are usually the result of a series of in-

dividual behaviors that seem to have no dramatic consequences at the moment we engage in each one of them.
People, for example, are often surprised to find themselves locked into jobs that they first envisaged as temporary. Accepting a pay raise, beginning to build an annuity,
taking an unexpected promotion, or relying on your sal-
ary to buy a new home may seem to be independent, dis-
crete decisions. Taken together, however, they can add up
to a career investment that seems impossible to reverse.
To use Becker's imagery, each apparently independent decision is like placing a brick in a wall that we are one day
shocked to learn has closed us in.

Surely Becker's description applies to all sorts of commitments. Here, the desperation that first leads people
into a medical culture with its drug treatments and corre-
sponding explanations for their difficulties is the beginning of a process of commitment that has far more wide-
ranging implications than people can possibly see at the
moment when they swallow the first pill prescribed for
them.

Experimentation

For the majority of those who use psychiatric drugs the
process involves trying many different medications over
time, each one beginning with the hope of success, but
then too often ending in disillusionment. The search for
the "right" drug is analogous to the search for Mr. or Ms.
Right. Just as people hold out hope of finding the perfect
mate despite repeated disappointments, those suffering

from depression often remain convinced that there's an ideal drug for them. One woman expressed the psychology behind experimentation:

> You sort of keep questioning yourself, why are you doing this. It's not helping. Some of it may actually be causing other problems, like problems sleeping. . . . But you know you sort of get invested in trying the medication. You've stepped over that threshold. And you know it's like, well, you might as well keep on going until you see if there's something that works. I was encouraged by the doctors, too. Not knowing anything about this journey, I just thought that this was what I was supposed to do. . . . But you start taking these medications and you sort of invest yourself in trying to find one that works. (female homemaker, aged 28)

A willingness to experiment, to throw oneself into the search for the medication that will finally do the trick, requires adopting a particular ideological perspective. Treatment with antidepressant medications is premised on the *assumption* that affective disorders are a consequence of neurotransmitter imbalances. Repeated often enough, the mantra of chemical imbalance becomes a kind of unassailable cultural fact. Recently at a meeting of my support group I collected a dozen or so informational brochures from drug companies. Each one told essentially the same scientific story as the one Pfizer offers to explain how its product Zoloft works: "*It is thought* that

Zoloft works by making serotonin more available where it is needed. This *may* help to correct the chemical imbalance that can cause depression. If your brain gets the right amount of serotonin, depression *might* improve" (my emphasis). To stick with drug experiments virtually requires the belief that your biology is bad:

> I would like people to know, "Don't be afraid to take a psychiatric drug. . . . Look at it as [though] it's a biochemical disorder. If you have bipolar disorder or unipolar disorder, what you're missing is the serotonin level in your blood. So you're taking this pill to make up for what you're missing." (female health advocate, aged 57)

> It's not the drugs. It's the illness which is so unpredictable. Because it can be strong when you're on meds, it can be weak when you're on meds. So I never look at the medication as the problem. It just isn't. It's the illness, that brain chemistry that goes awry. That's what causes my mental states. (female counselor, aged 59)

> Well, because it's a biochemical thing. It's like diabetes or high blood pressure. You can't cure yourself. You can deal with it and cope with it. I mean, type-two diabetes . . . I mean, I'll always be a diabetic. So yeah, I just feel that with a psychiatric illness you don't get cured from it. You learn how to cope with it. (female health advocate, aged 57)

> It is like something switched off in my mind. The volume was turned down, the static cleared. And that leads me to believe, obviously, that there is some kind of biological, organic basis to it. (salesman, aged 30)

While continuing the search for relief through medication requires at least a modicum of belief in biochemical causation, not everyone maintains equal faith in that explanation. Here the most appropriate analogy might be to religious belief systems. It would be hard to show up regularly to one's church, synagogue, or mosque without some degree of belief in the theology offered. At the same time, there is a continuum from true believers to skeptics. Moreover, faith is rarely constant. It waxes and wanes as believers confront the mysteries of the universe and the immediacy of events in their lives. In medicine, as in religion, thoughtful believers inevitably cope with uncertainty, confusion, and ambivalence about the veracity of their worldviews. In the end, most drug users combine biological and environmental explanations for their situation:

> I really believed that it . . . was a combination. That I had a [biological] inclination, and to boot I didn't have a very good childhood that made me feel confident and able to take on positive thinking about things. (female technical writer, aged 50)

> Perhaps I had a predisposition toward it [illness] genetically, and growing up in the chaos of New York

City and the hypocrisy . . . and just the constant motion and the constant bounce between up and down,
up and down in New York, you know, brought it out.
I don't think it's one thing or another. I think it can
be both. I think it rarely can be one. I don't think it's
only nature. I don't think it's only nurture. I think
it's both and I think that [pause]. I don't know, I
think that it's important to think about the way society . . . is constructing these diseases. (female graduate student, aged 29)

In the last chapter you heard Mike describe the tor-
tures of going up and down on different medications,
each of which had distinctive side effects. A few years ago
Peter Kramer, the author of *Listening to Prozac,* wrote a
book about human relationships entitled *Should You
Leave?*[4] The book explores perennially significant questions about intimacy and autonomy—"How do we choose
our partners? How well do we know them? How do mood
states affect our assessment of them and theirs of us?
When should we work to improve a relationship, and
when should we walk away?" In essence, Kramer could
have raised these same questions in his book on Prozac.
In the following instances, however, experiments were abject failures and the only real option was to walk away:

With the Zoloft, I would walk around with like a
sheet over me. Less sensation, less perception, less
cognition. You feel like, you got a 98, you got the
highest grade on a final. And I would be like, "Well,

that's good," and I'd go home and go to sleep for
twelve hours. I was tired all the time. I just felt like
nothing touched me. I wasn't sad, but I wasn't happy.
I just walked around and just blah all the time. I just
got used to it. . . . I didn't realize until I got off of it
what the drug was really doing to me. (female psychology student, aged 20)

I was a freak. I looked as if I were a freak. It was
parkinsonian. I had this involuntary neck spasm
which was, I believe . . . was from the imipramine—
the tricyclic. A person came into my office and said,
"Hi, good to see you, how you doing?" And I had this
involuntary movement. My head moved like an owl.
You know, 90 degrees. And I had no control of that
movement. I just had no control. I was seeing a doctor and I said, "I'm not taking this anymore. I can't
take it anymore. It's doing nothing for me." And I
think he might have recommended something else,
but I said nothing to him and wanted nothing to do
with medication. . . . Well, that was my first experience with medication—not a good experience. (male
media consultant, aged 52)

When I went on that fucking Neurontin, that's when
I got depressed. And I learned how to stay in bed all
day. I learned how to be depressed. . . . But I never
stayed in bed when I didn't have medication. You had
to get up and you had to go to work. I worked full

time. And you have to . . . live and, you know, you're
not gonna stop that. (female office worker, aged 60)

I do remember a small trial of Prozac. And all I remember is I didn't sleep at all for two days. None at
all. And I could hardly eat, and all I could do was cry.
And I got on a pay phone . . . and I said, "I want my
depression back. You know, get me off this." Another
doctor tried me on Elavil. And he must have put me
on a normal dose. . . . He prescribed Elavil and left
town. And I hallucinated on Elavil. . . . And I was
completely beside myself. I was numb. And I had to
get my husband's shrink to get me off of it. (female
writer, aged 59)

The notion of experimentation carries multiple meanings. On the one hand, those with whom I spoke were trying drugs as a possible way to minimize, ideally to escape,
their pain. Because antidepressant medications have such
wildly different effects on different individuals, doctors'
choice of medication for a patient clearly involves guesswork. When the result is "adverse reactions" to a string of
drugs, patients feel experimented *upon*. Several interviewees angrily described themselves as "guinea pigs." One
person complained, "I felt like he hung me out in the
wind. . . . He tried all those different drugs and none of
them worked and I just felt like a guinea pig or something." A woman who participated in a funded drug
study said, "As far as the psychiatric stuff, I think I've
been mostly a guinea pig, you know, a teaching tool."

As awful as these experiences are for people, perhaps worse still is the unfathomable disappointment they feel when a medication that temporarily "cured" them simply stops working. All psychotropic drugs can stop working even after a long period, sometimes years, of nearly unblemished success. When this happens, individuals can feel the sort of shock experienced when a lover suddenly leaves them:

> When I went to see the psychiatrist knowing that he would probably put me on an antidepressant . . . [I was feeling] very hopeful, thinking that I was going to have a normal life. [I was going to] get back to work, get back to functioning well. Taking the amitriptyline, having it work fairly well . . . then having it poop out. That's a blow. I can remember the first week that happened, and that was seventeen years ago. (unemployed male, aged 51)

The kind of early drug experimentation described in this section is premised on the expectation of cure. While only a few people in my sample talked of having been cured, nearly all came to realize that their drugs were going to work imperfectly. Most of the interviewees slowly recognized that mental illness is a permanent condition and that there is no easy fix. Still, there must be a moment somewhere along the way when a patient acknowledges that the problem is unlikely ever fully to disappear. That moment, no doubt, constitutes an epiphany, albeit a negative one, that sets in motion a whole new view of their relationship with medication.

Engagement

An engaged couple has to confront many real-life decisions that are rarely a part of early courtship. They must work out agreements about such matters as money, mutual obligations, a division of family labor, and power. The kind of escalating commitment represented by an engagement calls forth more serious and sustained efforts to concretize the couple's "joint reality," a process that can become difficult and contentious. To be sure, once we have made a more solid commitment to *any* relationship, we must more intensively work out the likely form of the relationship over the long term. Each time we raise the commitment ante, we start a new round of reality testing and negotiation.

Having decided to begin taking medication and then having passed through initial stages of drug trials, most people reach a critical point in their medication careers. They are unlikely to forswear medication if it has helped them significantly. For the majority of those I interviewed, deciding whether to continue taking medication was a difficult process. Realizing that they were in a far-from-perfect relationship, they expressed commitment phobia. Family, friends, and doctors were telling them they would be far better off if they would only stick with their medications. Like those described in self-help books such as Rhonda Findling's *The Commitment Cure: What to*

Do When You Fall for an Ambivalent Man, many alternated between splitting up with medications and embracing them.[5]

> It's [depression] just being dealt with because of the pill. I'd much rather learn to deal with it [myself] because it's a part of me. Depression is a huge part of my life. It's one of the big issues since I was eleven. I went back on [the pills] again. I'd been off them for two weeks. I was getting worse and worse and I went back on them a couple of days ago. It's an experiment that will continue to fail, I think, for the rest of my life. I think I'm never going to be completely off pills. (female drama student, aged 19)

> I guess I wanted to see if I could be normal, if I could just put the past behind me and move forward and not have this extra complication in my life. I know that I'd just rather not be dependent on anything. . . . I mean, maybe that's . . . why I get rid of the drugs every now and then. . . . I guess I keep hoping that there's going to be some time when I don't need anything, when I can just sort of get through the bumps of life and have that be my life. (female homemaker, aged 28)

> And I've tried to be the person that I am on the drugs, without them. But I can't do it. Over the last ten years [I've tried to stop] hundreds of times. I've

> tried going completely pill-less. And it doesn't work
> out very well for me. (female accountant, aged 29)

Stopping and starting medications is one way people avoid commitment and try to regain control of their lives. However, since the people I interviewed had typically been using psychotropic medications for years, they represented a segment of the drug-taking population that had remained relatively committed to a medical model of mental illness. In the middle of their drug careers most still envisioned a time when they would stop taking medication. Quitting remained a long-term goal for them. For the time being, though, they had come to feel that, all things considered, they were better off with their medications. They had decided that their drug relationship, with all its flaws, was worth retaining. At that point they became more deeply engaged with pharmacological treatments and thus more active participants in their own care. Previously the passive objects of doctors' experiments, those who decide to continue using medication become proactive experimenters. They may also demand a more democratic and mutually respectful relationship with their physicians:

> The medication only works . . . because of the doctor
> who is giving it to me and the way we work together.
> . . . I am a well-read patient and know about this
> stuff, my psychiatrist respects me and will say, "Well,
> what do you think we should do now?" . . . She takes

my recommendations to heart, doesn't just say, "Oh yeah, whatever, tough luck, you're taking this." There are never any ultimatums. (female graduate student, aged 29)

The second doctor . . . insisted on prescribing 300 milligrams of trazodone to help me sleep. Yet she would tell me if you can't sleep after taking 300, after twenty minutes take a fourth [pill]. So at the end of the month, inevitably I'd have to call her up and say I need another few more pills. . . . So then after a while she starts barking at me because I'm requesting more pills. And it's not my fault. I mean, I need them. . . . And [finally] I told her I didn't want her as my doctor anymore. . . . She was out. She was definitely out. (unemployed female, aged 58)

During the writing of this book my son became engaged. He had been going out with his fiancée for quite some time, and they had been living together for well over a year before he proposed marriage. After the happy announcement I asked him why it had taken so long to make a firm commitment. He explained that they had first to work out some issues. When I asked for examples, he mentioned such things as the amount of time he might spend alone with male friends, how they would balance their work and their life together, and how they would manage money. Like other engaged couples, my son and my future daughter-in-law had to work out thorny questions around personal autonomy and control in their relationship.

Such issues may persist throughout a marriage, but they are likely to be most intense as partners are deciding on the permanence of their commitment. In the same way, those who have decided to remain on medication feel the need to exercise autonomy and control. One way to do so is to make independent decisions about dosage:

Well, they [parents] would ask if I had taken my pills [that day]. And I would say yes. And a lot of the time I knew they would find out that I hadn't. (female sociology student, aged 20)

I guess I felt proud of myself too that I didn't have to wait for someone to tell me [to cut back]; to have this whole sort of interaction and decision-making process. . . . And it was just much easier just to do it by myself and to at least try to see what would happen. (female homemaker, aged 28)

I guess what I feel is that it's okay to take medication, but I would like to take as little as possible, and I would like to keep at that edge. I would like to risk being a little upset and be there [rather than feeling drugged]. There was a Tuesday night that I was exhausted and I thought, "I wonder if I can sleep without this stuff." And I did it. I went to sleep and I stayed asleep and I woke up and I was me! (female office worker, aged 60)

Once people have made the fundamental decision to continue on medications, the question becomes how best to live with their new partner; how to reach accommodations that will make the relationship healthy and satisfying. The shift in emphasis from "whether" to "how best" to maintain a medication relationship solidifies their investment in the biomedical model of mental illness and its claim to appropriate treatments. While many may still dream about a future free of pills, by this point they have likely made a lifelong commitment to drug therapy. The decisive moment comes with the realization that "I've accepted now that this is the way I am. This [using medications] is what I'll need to do *for the rest of my life.*"

Marriage

Although most of the people I interviewed were hesitant to commit to a long-term relationship with medications, life with drugs had typically become a routine part of their existence. Despite misgivings about long-term use of antidepressants, most had come to believe that they were better off with them than without them. Over time they had become wedded to a biomedical version of mental illness that solidified their relationship to medication:

> I am very, very grateful for what the drugs have done
> to me, regardless of the fact that I am treatment resis-
> tant and . . . it's constantly shifting, and all of that.
> And I probably will be addicted to some kind of
> [benzodiazepine] for the rest of my life. And I still . . .

hate it sometimes. I want to throw them all out the window . . . but I have nothing else to put my faith in. (female graduate student, aged 29)

I'll take whatever I have to take. I'll deal with whatever side effects there are. Life goes on. (female counselor, aged 59)

I think I'll always regret having started medication even for any of the good that it did in my life. To not know what I could do on my own without it is very difficult. I mean, there was a sort of deterioration of that resolve in me to get through anything when I started taking drugs. I sort of felt like, "Well, gee, now that I'm sick, it's okay to be sick," you know, that there's something that I don't have to fight through anymore. There's a reason and it's not that I can't do something or I'm too lazy or whatever. But there was something in me that gave up the fight. (female homemaker, aged 28)

There's still a part of me that wishes I wouldn't have to take them for the rest of my life, but you know, I will have to take them for the rest of my life and that's fine with me. (retired female office worker, aged 56)

I have spoken about the way many of my interviewees ultimately capitulated to the idea that they would have to take pills for the rest of their lives. Others described themselves as surrendering, yielding, or giving up when they finally arrived at the realization that their relationship with medications was a lifelong commitment. To even out the picture, I should note that for some of the people I spoke with the decision to stay on medication was far more positive. For them medication had been beneficial if not literally lifesaving. They embraced their drug relationships and could not imagine ever being without them:

> I'm going to stay on my medication. I have no plans to ever go off the medication. I don't see any reason why I should. It took so long to finally get to the right meds. I'm really happy with what's going on right now. (female health advocate, aged 57)

> [Nardil] was just a miracle. I always had this strange sense of like I had just gone through World War III and the world somehow was different. It was that I was different, but it felt like the world was. . . . There were times when I really felt good and then I felt pretty much back to normal. And I thought that I was out of the woods. As far as my relationship with the Nardil, I saw this pill work. . . . It was like in the textbooks. . . . Within a few weeks suddenly I had a response. And so ever since then my feeling has been there is nothing that I would do to put myself in the position of being that sick again. If that meant taking drugs, even dangerous ones like Nardil, for the rest of my life, I would do it. . . . I mean it [the illness]

practically destroyed my life. (male physician,
aged 44)

I'm enhancing what I already have by taking medication. I'm going to complete the whole process by taking the medication. So it becomes this maturing process. . . . In the beginning being so resistant to taking
it . . . [resistant] to trying all these different things
and not committing to anything because I don't
know who I am or who they are. And as you become a
little bit more comfortable with where you are and
who you are, it becomes much easier to find a com-
plement to that or something that will complete
what else is there. It really completes a process that
wouldn't be completed unless I had the medication.
So . . . I was desperate and didn't have anything else
to do. And even though nothing else before worked,
this is going to be the best thing. This is going to be
the best thing to complete this whole piece. . . . I'm
not ready to pull the plug to try something else. I
mean, who wants to mess around with what works? If
it works, you're going to keep it. (female sociology
student, aged 20)

I wouldn't want to stop. I feel like they're [drugs] a
part of my life. (female administrative aide, aged 54)

Relationships are bounded by behaviors that become
taken-for-granted, routine dimensions of daily life constructed over a long period of time. Indeed, this chapter

has been about the process through which initially dramatic decisions in a person's life can over time become nearly as commonplace as breathing. Taking psychiatric medications—once the source of great anguish—can become emotionally equivalent to taking vitamin pills or brushing one's teeth before bedtime:

> There came a time last year when I went into my therapist's office, and that was the first time when I woke up and . . . didn't think of myself as being ill. And so at this point I don't wake up and think of myself being ill. It doesn't cross through my mind.

> *Well, what do you think about when you take your Topamax? What do you think when you open the bottle?*

> I don't know. I don't think it crosses my mind. I mean, I just open the bottle and take them. I don't really think about anything. I mean, I'm rushing around my room getting ready for class, and then as I go to bed I just take another one. I've got to take them like I take a vitamin or anything else.

> *So you've reached the point where you see it in the category of vitamins?*

> Well, I don't think they're in the category of vitamins, but I still know what it's there for. But I don't think of it like, "Oh, it's for mental illness." . . . I just take it without thinking about what it is. (female psychology student, aged 21)

Commitments are double-edged. They have the potential both to enhance identities and to threaten them. A life without commitments to work, to places, to causes, to ideas, and to others is hard to imagine. Others define us and we define ourselves by the ties we construct. By contrast, ties may become so tightly binding and consuming that they cause us to lose sight of who we really are. Over time some commitments can feel stifling, thus undermining our sense of authenticity. Perhaps the identity tensions posed by commitments are especially evident in the United States, given its ethic of individualism. Americans simultaneously believe in personal freedom and crave the intimacy, community, and comfort of deep connections.

Love and relationship commitments illustrate this duality well. On the one hand we celebrate the joy of giving ourselves fully, freely, and completely to another person. Wedding vows center on the promise to love, honor, and cherish one's partner in sickness and in health, in good times and in bad, and until the end of one's life. The vast majority of Americans marry at some point in their lives believing that they can fully realize who they are only through love and commitment. On the other hand, partners in a marriage often come to feel that their own interests, needs, and goals have become compromised by the very commitments they initially thought would complete them. A sense of self-loss no doubt contributes to the failure of nearly half of all marriages in the United States.

Just as the commitments required by love create identity dilemmas, so do those required by a full commitment to a biomedical version of the causes and proper treatments for affective disorders. While several people joyfully told me that their medications allowed them to discover at last the person they were meant to be, others expressed distress about losing a sense of self as a consequence of using psychotropic medications. In both cases, the process of committing to medication necessarily involves a radical transformation of self.

Chapter 4

Searching for Authenticity

Every morning when I . . . take the medication, I feel like I'm
putting on my lifejacket for the day and I can just bob in the
ocean. I'm not flying into the sky. I'm not lifting off. . . . And
when I'm just bobbing in the ocean . . . I don't feel like I'm
living. . . . I don't feel like I have an identity.

—male peace activist,

aged 22

Questions about personal authenticity surround us these days and have become a matter of public discourse. Some political pundits have suggested that George W. Bush's appeal to millions of voters was his down-home, unpretentious self. With Bush you presumably get what you see. For many of those same people John Kerry seemed inauthentic. Was he just "one of the guys," as portrayed in a photo-op hunting expedition, or was he really the elite preppy who preferred wind-surfing in designer gear? In a culture obsessed with celebrity and fame, tabloids draw audiences with revealing stories about what their favorite stars are really like.[1] More to the point of this book, the world of sports has been turned upside down by recent scandals involving suspected steroid use among high-achieving athletes. In the private realm, women whose partners use Viagra have expressed concern that the quality of their intimate relations is less related to their attractiveness than to the effects of a pill.

The connections among new medical technologies, authenticity, and identity have attracted the attention of medical ethicists and philosophers.[2] At the center of the debate is the blurry distinction between medical therapies and medical "enhancements." Increasingly, medical technologies and pharmaceuticals are used to help healthy people "change for the better." For example, some argue that psychotropic medications are justifiably used by people who are not suffering from significant emotional illnesses. By allowing people to become less shy, less sensitive, or less plagued by small worries, advocates claim, the medications may help them discover their real selves. Opponents have a less benign view about the morality of enhancement technologies:

> When a person undergoes surgery so that she can speak like a woman, or changes her nose with cosmetic surgery, or takes an anti-depressant that transforms her from a shrinking violet to the life of the party, what is at issue is not simply whether the change is for the better or for the worse, or even whether the change has been mediated by technology, but the mere fact that the person has changed. She may not have exactly become a "different person,"

even in a figurative sense, but her identity may well
have changed in a way that would strike many of us
as morally significant. . . . Our ambivalence about so
many enhancement technologies is often ambivalence about the kinds of people we want to be.[3]

While none of the people I interviewed for this book
were using psychiatric medications simply to enhance
otherwise healthy selves, they were nevertheless clearly
changed by the drugs they were taking. Almost to a person they felt that medication made them different. While
such transformations may occasionally raise moral questions, they almost always provoke puzzling questions
about identity and authenticity. Whatever their life circumstances, every human being wonders, at some point,
"Who am I really? Is there an essential self that distinguishes me from others? How does my sense of self
change over time?" To complicate the matter, perhaps we
have as many selves as there are situations in which we
act.[4]

Psychiatric drugs add another layer to the search for
self because they influence our feelings and moods. They
alter our consciousness, and in doing so, they potentially
refashion who we believe ourselves to be. To the degree
that we associate ourselves with our feelings—we are, in
large measure, what we feel—it should come as no surprise that drug-induced changes in feelings can arouse
substantial reflection about selves gained and lost.

Drugs, like all objects, assume meanings that are socially imposed, vary across groups and cultures, and

change over time. And yet contemporary medicine, based on rational, scientific principles, largely restricts its purview to the biological effects of medications on body cells. It fails to consider the ways psychotropic drugs affect the identities of those who use them. To varying degrees, taking antidepressants required all the people I interviewed to think about three issues: (1) whether they were ready to cross what they viewed as a significant identity boundary; (2) what it means to feel like oneself; and (3) whether one's "true" self is revealed or obscured by the pills one takes. To the extent that psychiatric drug use poses fundamental questions about identity, it can shed light on how all of us understand who we are at our core.

Crossing Identity Boundaries

Among the people I interviewed were several who sought drug treatment from the onset of their illness, who welcomed the relief that they thought psychiatric drugs would provide, or who were so desperate that they would do anything to escape the pain of depression. We might well expect that as drug companies market their products more widely, more people will actively seek them out. To be sure, the explosive growth of psychotropic drug use suggests that an increasing number of Americans see pills as an appropriate response to a wide array of human problems. At the same time, most of the people in my sample were resistant to medication, at least initially. Over and again, they expressed a deep reluctance to take medication despite the urging of friends, family, and physicians. To take a pill was to cross an important identity line.

One young woman used the metaphor of crossing a threshold to describe her decision to take medications for the first time. Andrea was a graduate student in social work preparing for an administrative career. She recalled the emotions stirred up when she had stood in front of the hospital doors, deciding whether to keep a medical appointment that would almost certainly lead to a prescription for an antidepressant medication. In her case literally walking into the hospital carried enormous symbolic weight. She recognized that entering the hospital meant initiating a drug career and a dramatic shift in identity:

> Just opening the doors was a big deal. Going from just the outside air to the inside air . . . You know what distinguished me from the people standing outside smoking? Hovering on the edges of the external world versus the world [beyond the doors] . . . it was like a lump in my throat. It was just a sort of semi-paralysis where I would just sort of have to steel myself to get through the couple of feet up the stairs to the doorway . . . and walk through. And then when I was through, it was a whole other thing. Then there was like these doctors walking around. And it was very easy to distinguish who was sick and who wasn't, or at least who had the role of being sick and who had the role of being the professional, by the way that

they dressed or acted or what they [said]. And I
looked more the role of the professional. And you
know, it was a very weird place to be. . . . I had started
the master's program by then. And it was very difficult . . . just sort of straddling the line between "Hey,
I'm going to be someone who's going to be taking
care of other people or trying to make the world a
better place through my profession, and yet I am . . .
or could potentially become as sick as these people
standing here. And what's the difference? What's the
difference between the two realities? Which person
am I? Am I the sick person or am I the professional?"

Here is how a teacher described his fears about taking
the first pill:

I remember when I was about to take my first pill. I
. . . was determined I was going to take it that hour or
that evening. [I was a] little bit bathed in self-pity, almost. Poor Frank, you're losing part of yourself. Part
of yourself is being taken away from you because you
have to take this medicine. Isn't this too bad that you
have whatever you have because it means you have to
take this pill and you're losing part of yourself. . . . It
was the fact of being altered. Now I'm no longer going to be who I was. Because these chemicals do
something and so [there is] this notion of integrity of
a human being, of how everything interacts. . . .
When you take these pills [you] somehow alter the
structure inside you, which is not a simple structure.

And [it's a structure] which we don't know [much
about]. . . . I was losing part of myself.

Most of my interviewees who initially resisted taking
medication were afraid of being labeled mentally ill. The
following words express this common theme:

I think I had ambivalent feelings about medications.
So many people I knew were on them, or had been on
them, that it wasn't completely stigmatized, a stigmatizing experience for me. . . . Yeah, it was '92, so
Prozac had been out for, whatever, three or four or
five years. [But] I felt like it was serious. I thought of
it as more serious, as a step toward something worse.
(female graduate student, aged 29)

Part of me still didn't want to accept or had a hard
time accepting that I was . . . I had a mental illness.
That I was depressed enough . . . clinically that someone was wanting to have me try certain medications
to alleviate the illness, you know—the mental illness,
not the physical illness. . . . It's very confusing. I think
the whole experience . . . you sort of keep questioning
yourself why are you doing this. (female homemaker,
aged 28)

People do not understand that . . . it's not just taking
a pill. There's a lot more to it than that. It's not just
taking a pill and ending depression, you're dealing
with a whole mental thing, too. . . . [You're] being la-

beled, taking Zoloft and being labeled [as] someone
who takes medicine. There's just a lot to deal with.
(male education student, aged 20)

Many expressed the feeling that a diagnosis of mental
illness and the suggestion that they take medications
made them feel "defective":

> I had been diagnosed when I was twelve with bipolar.
> I had been hospitalized twice. I had a suicide attempt
> at twelve. And so it was already known. It was already
> labeled there's something just wrong with her.
> There's just something wrong with her . . . and it just
> spilled into everything. It was in the context espe-
> cially within my family, but I think it spilled . . . into
> relationships and because there really was something
> fundamentally wrong with me. I wasn't fixable. I
> wasn't changeable. You talk about an identity, but it's
> just an identity of yuckiness. (female sociology stu-
> dent, aged 20)

The symbolic importance of doctor-prescribed pill-taking as a kind of identity point of no return is powerfully
illustrated by Sarah's case. Recall from Chapter 3 that
Sarah's persistent insomnia had caused her, in her own
words, to abuse over-the-counter remedies for many years.
However, she had steadfastly refused to visit a psychiatrist or to take prescribed medications. Then, after her
mother's death, she had found a large stockpile of Xanax,
a powerful antianxiety drug, among her mother's belong-

ings. She had begun using the pills liberally, until eventually she became dependent on them. Even with this long history of drug use, however, she resisted the idea of taking pills prescribed by a doctor:

> I did go to the doctor when I was in my early thirties. And I said, "You know, I can't sleep. I get very anxious. . . ." He said, "I am giving you a prescription for Valium." I didn't want to take it. . . . To me it would be like labeling me that I needed a prescription for Valium. . . . [But] the over-the-counter thing was something I [could do]. You know, if I were just messing around with over-the-counter stuff [I was okay]. . . . I always entertained the thought that by doing the over-the-counter thing I could stop whenever I wanted to.

At first Sarah's thinking seems paradoxical. She freely consumes large volumes of pills found on pharmacy shelves and then becomes hooked on a drug prescribed for someone else. At the same time, she refuses to accept her doctor's recommendation that she take a minor tranquilizer. Perhaps, though, her behavior makes more sense when viewed in the context of a general cultural ambivalence about whether we should each be in control of our emotions. As long as Sarah resists the patient role by treating herself, she maintains at least the illusion of personal control over her feelings and, thus, responsibility for them.

The society in which we live offers contradictory messages about personal responsibility.[5] On the one hand, the biomedical model of mental illness as a product of broken brains is welcome because it relieves people of responsibility for their circumstances. On the other hand, relieving people of responsibility for how they feel can result in a sense of powerlessness. One man I interviewed captured the paradox :

> You talk about personal identity. The good news is
> that it's biogenic [and] therefore it's not my fault.
> The bad news is it's biogenic because I'm just a pas-
> senger on life's way, and I have no idea of who's driv-
> ing me where and to what destination.

Despite the popularity of biological explanations for mental illness, as a society we expect people to manage their emotions, and we have very little tolerance for those who cannot.[6] For example, even in clear instances of crimes committed during psychotic episodes, the insanity defense rarely works in the American legal system. In the end, we expect people to be responsible for themselves and to work through their problems. With remarkable regularity the people I interviewed expressed uneasiness about controlling their feelings with a pill. The notion that one ought to "tough it out" without medication is evident in these remarks:

> I didn't want to rely on something to make me feel
> better. I'm supposed to do it by myself because I'm
> a human being. Everyone else can do it by themselves,
> so why can't I? (female sociology student, aged 20)

> This [depression] is always going to be a part of my
> life. . . . It's never going to go away, but I have to just
> deal with it. . . . Can I ever feel that bad again? Proba-
> bly, and I can recognize it all now. And I think that I
> can handle it. I will handle it without medication. It's
> not an option for me right now. I would go to some-
> thing of a natural . . . going to herbs or something
> like that before I ever go to [medication]. . . . And be-
> ing dependent on a drug. I do not like having to be
> dependent on something like that. (female market re-
> searcher, aged 35)

As these accounts show, people's self-esteem and sense of integrity are deeply connected to their ability to control their personal problems. The people I spoke with had difficulty accepting fully the idea that emotional illnesses are no different from physiological problems such as heart disease or diabetes. It may be comforting to hear that antidepressant medications correct chemical imbalances in the brain just as insulin controls diabetes. But most of those I interviewed assigned different meanings to mental and physical conditions. When asked directly, they affirmed that psychiatric drugs are far more likely than other medications to make them feel bad about themselves:

> It's a different species of being. It is the magical
> thinking that I will be this . . . that whatever is caus-
> ing these instabilities and these tremendous mood
> swings will eventually be set on the right course. I

won't have to think about taking medications that
serve as a constant reminder that I have this psychiatric illness . . . which is stigmatizing. (male media consultant, aged 52)

I tried at least two well-known antidepressants before
getting to the Wellbutrin. There may have even been
another one before that too. I mean, it was not a fun
journey because you go to this doctor and you sort of
expect that "Oh, they're going to give you this medication." And unfortunately it's not like an antibiotic
where you've been diagnosed and you have an ear infection, that you have some sort of infection and
here's the medication from the doctor. It's a little
script that looks like any other script, except that it
says psychiatric on it, which really weirded me out for
a while to take that to a pharmacist. (female homemaker, aged 28)

My conversations also revealed that resistance to psychiatric medications is tied up in complex ways with
people's feelings about altering their minds and brains.
Although many classes of medication affect brain chemistry, there is something especially frightening about using
drugs that "mess around with my brain":

You want to be normal. Why be dependent on this
damn pill? My brain is . . . I could do things with my
brain that many people can't do. And why does my
brain now or whatever need a chemical to make me

somewhat normal? And it was an awful battle for years. Also, I had to decide the difference between—in my mind—medication and a mind-altering drug. I had to bounce . . . those two terms back and forth. A medication is something that is helpful. A mind-altering drug changes your personality. And that was the way I was feeling. (retired small-business owner, aged 68)

The fact that I was going to take something that would affect my mind . . . was very scary to me. I mean, talk about your feeling of losing control. They are powerful drugs, and it was frightening to me that I was going to go in and mess around with my mind. It was very scary. . . . That's my life up there. So it was scary to me. (female technical writer, aged 50)

To be sure, antidepressants do alter brain chemistry and thereby affect feelings, perceptions, thoughts, and moods. Virtually everyone in my sample continued to question how psychotropic medications affect who they are at their core. But the eradication of painful symptoms can also call forth questions about what constitutes one's self.

Feeling Like Oneself

In the first chapter I mentioned Lauren Slater's memoir, *Prozac Diary*. Recall Slater's description of how Prozac liberated her from crushing depression and debilitating obsessive-compulsive behaviors. Although her worst symptoms had virtually disappeared with medication, Slater did not feel like her "self" and struggled with the decision to stay on the drug. In another extraordinary memoir, Kay Redfield Jamison similarly described the loss of self spawned by "normalcy":

> Moods are such an essential part of the substance of life, of one's notion of oneself. . . . In my case, I had a horrible sense of loss for who I had been and where I had been. It was difficult to give up the high flights of mind and mood, even though the depressions that inevitably followed nearly cost me my life. . . . My family and friends expected that I would welcome being "normal," be appreciative of lithium, and take in stride having normal energy and sleep. . . . People say when I complain of being less lively, less energetic, less high-spirited, "Well, now you're just like the rest of us," meaning, among other things, to be reassuring. But I compare myself with my former self, not with others. Not only that, I tend to compare my current self with the best I have been, which is when I have been mildly manic. When I am my present "normal" self, I am far removed from when I have been my liveliest, most productive, most intense, most outgoing and effervescent. In short, for myself, I am a hard act to follow.[7]

Like Slater and Jamison, several people I interviewed reported that medication miraculously restored them to "normalcy." The interviews contain comments like these: "He gave me amitriptyline, which is . . . supposed to take two weeks to six weeks to work. It took two weeks [and] I felt like a brand-new person." "And sure enough within four or five weeks I started . . . even before that, maybe a week or two, I started feeling well." "When you find one that works, for the period of time when it's working, it's worth its weight in gold and platinum." As the last comment suggests, medication miracles are too often short-lived, although many individuals did experience significant long-term relief from their symptoms. People struggled to explain some of the subtle ways in which the medications dulled feelings they greatly valued. Often the descriptions they offered were simultaneously distressing and uplifting. A doctor spoke of "finding my eyes again" (that is, having courage to tell people what he really feels) while losing the capacity to feel appropriate sadness:

> I've lost tears. I heard something on the radio and it
> clearly reminded me of my mother, some early stuff
> that she would sing to me from the song "Lightly
> Like a Rose." . . . I was at [the] cemetery taking a
> walk. It was a beautiful morning. The lilacs were out.
> The lilies of the valley that my mother loved were out.
> Everything was really nice, and on the radio was . . . a
> jazz piano player, sweetly playing "Lightly Like a
> Rose," [and it] immediately caught me. And I listened
> to it. I wanted to cry. I just couldn't do it. It was clear
> that the trough had been cut off. And I knew, and I
> knew that it was the Prozac. . . . And I said, "Fuck

you, Prozac, I want to cry for my mom." (male physician, aged 54)

Or consider the case of a young man who could not decide his feelings for the women he was dating:

> The other thing is that it really impacts my identity, because I feel like I'm still developing who I am, and I haven't figured out my basic personality. I haven't figured out what I want in life, in a partner, in what kind of girl I'm looking for. And sometimes I feel like the depression and the medication and feeling better confuses that. . . . I mean, I've been trying to date a few girls recently. And I also think part of the medication's impact on me is that I don't know how I'm feeling. I always second-guess how I'm feeling emotionally about another person. It's a flat line. I don't have real joy. But when I feel sad and I feel like I should be depressed about something, I'm not. When I feel like I'm trying to figure out if I really like somebody, if I maybe love them, I can't figure that out, because I don't have those feelings. . . . When you're on medication that's part of the second-guessing. So you don't know if that's you or if that's the drug. (male peace activist, aged 22)

As the last quote suggests, the significance given to medications varies not only over the course of an illness but also with the moment the illness is experienced in the life course of the individual. The meanings attached to psychiatric drug use are simply not the same for a child diagnosed at age eleven, a teenager, a young adult establishing intimate ties, a middle-aged person, or a senior citizen. Indeed, as we enter different stages of development we incorporate new feelings into our emotional repertoire.[8] Affective disorders can compromise human development because, by definition, they distort "normal" feelings. However, we must also consider the possibility that psychotropic medications, by limiting the range of feelings a person can experience, may equally impact emotional development.

Thus far, the people we have heard in this section have been commenting on the relatively subtle ways medications have changed their feelings. Sometimes the connections between drug use and emotional changes are unclear. In other cases, however, alterations in moods, feelings, and emotions are sufficiently intense after taking a medication that there is no mistaking cause. The drug then has two opposing effects: desirable feelings are either gained or lost. Drug success stories center on the eradication of unwanted feelings and the availability of feelings that make life more manageable:

> I've had one fabulous reaction. I took Celexa and I was happy and I was laughing. And it wasn't like sarcastic, you know—I'm very sarcastic and I enjoy sarcasm and dry humor and I'll laugh at that. But it was like laughing and I walked down the street, and if I see someone whistling or hear someone whistling . . . to me someone whistling is symbolic of this happi-

ness that I want to achieve. And I can remember what it's like. People don't whistle if they're depressed. You know, nobody depressed is walking around the street whistling. You don't whistle unless you are like psyched and you are loving life. . . . And when I was on Celexa, it was just . . . my sister described it as just this person who she always knew I was but was just underneath everything. And she just felt so happy that I was able to come out, and I just felt like this freedom. . . . And my depression is always just weighing me down and [now] . . . it was a freedom and a lightness. And I could go to the gym because I was light enough. It was . . . there was nothing weighing me down. [long pause] Sometimes I feel like that, you know, without being on Celexa or without being on medication, but it's very fleeting. And I'd like to think that I am the person who I was on Celexa. (female psychology student, aged 20)

Psychiatric drugs typically have more mixed results, however. They are clearly a powerful tool for relieving extreme depression or mania, but the relief is too often partial and inconsistent. Frequently, it also comes at a heavy price. Many people told me they felt robbed of feelings that were central to their view of themselves. Even when the medications "worked" they repeatedly complained that they had lost important parts of themselves:

I think there is a definitely serious identity question. I don't feel like the same person on drugs. I feel as though maybe I'm a better person, but it's not who I am. . . . I mean, maybe you might get to see the bad side [without medications], but that's still part of who I am, you know, the bad side. It's an identity issue to me, I think. (male education student, aged 20)

I'm a complicated person and it's a difficult life and I make mistakes. But I'm there and then I take the pills, and my therapist told me that the pills would make me more like me. . . . I go back to her and I say, "It's not happening." You know, the pills take me away from me, they do something else. The lithium sort of organizes me, the Wellbutrin lifts me up, the Benadryl puts me down. But it's not me. (female office worker, aged 60)

It's possible that the reason for my slowness getting going in the mornings . . . is because of what I'm on now. That may be [the case] and it may be too [big] a price to pay . . . for relative peace of mind [during] the other parts of the day. But on . . . other drugs and at other times . . . I couldn't think. I couldn't even drive. I wasn't me. And that's a horrible feeling. And it's terrible to have to choose between not being you on a drug and a terrible depression. (female writer, aged 59)

The dilemma of having to choose between a measure of wellness and significant loss of self is most clearly evident and profoundly felt when a drug's side effects interfere with important aspects of one's identity. The inserts that accompany psychiatric drug prescriptions leave no doubt that, like all powerful drugs, they can cause a wide range of side effects. Among the side effects most frequently mentioned by interviewees as too big a price even for wellness were weight gain and sexual dysfunction.[9] One woman, who went from 140 pounds to 250 pounds within a matter of months, said:

> Well, what happened when I was on Zyprexa and Clozaril was I was finally happy. I finally had relief of my symptoms. . . . But I also had no clue how far it was going to go before I recognized I didn't look like myself anymore. I looked in the mirror and felt like an alien. I felt like I was no longer a woman. I didn't feel the same way sexually with men. I didn't feel the same.

Although drug companies generally claim that a small percentage of those taking SSRIs experience sexual dysfunction, clinicians routinely report that as many as 50 to 60 percent of their patients, both men and women, experience disturbing sexual difficulties.[10] One woman said: "I don't know if it's the worst effect, but one of the effects was that you don't feel sexual, you don't feel your own sexuality or you don't look at anybody. Nobody looks attractive." And one man described the Hobson's choice so many face between psychological pain and side effects that erode fundamental identities:

So I see this doctor and you know, the first thing he says is he gives me Prozac and we talked about sexual dysfunction. And I said to him, "You know something," I said, "I'm not sure that the cure isn't worse than the illness that's being treated here because I'm dead from the waist down." Before I was dead from the waist up [and] now from the waist down. I said, "What's left? Do you think that's going to elevate my mood that I can no longer function sexually?" I was literally dead and it wasn't doing anything to my mood. So Prozac was out of the question. Then we moved to Zoloft. (male media consultant, aged 52)

In *Prozac Diary* Lauren Slater observes that though a great deal has been written about what happens to people when they become sick, very little has been said about the equally powerful consequences of becoming well. Like the inmates portrayed in the movie *The Shawshank Redemption* who cannot deal with freedom after decades of institutionalization, some of my interviewees found it difficult to contemplate—and sometimes live—a life free of depression or mania. They missed their illness because it is who they fundamentally define themselves to be. While the vast majority of those who suffer from affective disorders choose pills over pain, the choice is not as easy as one might imagine:

I always had these very deep feelings, and I used to write poetry to express how I felt. On medication, I'm not so hot to do that. And so I think it does take a piece away from me, a more poetic and maybe creative part of me. And that's another one of those trade-offs. . . . I notice when I'm off the Celexa . . . I just sometimes feel things so acutely. . . . I think I was born this way. I have a very strong empathetic streak. I don't always like those feelings because they're uncomfortable. . . . I guess it's all about tolerating feelings. Can I tolerate the feelings that feel bad to me in order to experience . . . who I am? These drugs are wonderful and can really help a person, but . . . there is a compromise there. (female technical writer, aged 50)

Before I went on medication, all I wanted was to be able to go out with my friends and go to a bar and be able to sit there and spend the time, because before I would be scared to get on the train. I would be fearful of going out, and once I was there I would have to leave after a short while. And now I can. I can go out and I have a life and I enjoy it. But sometimes I feel I really, really, miss that spiritual side of me. And it was becoming a major part of my identity and who I was, and how it was going to shape my life and how I was going to live my life. (male peace activist, aged 22)

In an earlier book, *The Burden of Sympathy,* I explored the effects of mental illness on those who care for sick family members.[11] I found that parents, spouses, children, and siblings struggle to honor commitments to a loved one without becoming engulfed by that person's misery. Many caregivers acknowledged sometimes feeling strongly negative emotions—even hate—toward a family member they are supposed to love. Most, however, quickly amended their "confession" by distinguishing between the individual and the illness. It was, they explained, really the illness that deserved their anger, not the person. Still, it was a source of troubling ambivalence that caregivers could never be certain just how to separate the person from the illness.

People suffering from depression may also have difficulty understanding whether their troubles arise from their illness or from some independent, core self. Those with a long history of psychiatric drug use face an additional challenge—to distinguish the pill from the person. That is, after years of drug-taking, most of those I interviewed longed to know who they would be in the absence of the drugs. Even those who felt well, even cured, on their medications often fiddled with dosage levels and considered stopping their medication altogether. For many, the urge to know one's own true self prompted ongoing experimentation with medications.

Searching for a True Self

Because psychiatric medications are designed to change moods, feelings, and behaviors, people taking them for prolonged periods of time often begin to wonder: *Is this me or is it the drug?* No one can know for sure. As the Czech writer Milan Kundera expressed so eloquently in his novel *The Unbearable Lightness of Being*, the human condition makes such existential doubt all but inevitable: "We can never know what to want, because, living only one life, we can neither compare it with our previous lives nor perfect it in our lives to come. . . . There is no means of testing which decision is better, because there is no basis for comparison. We live everything as it comes, without warning, like an actor going on cold."[12] This dilemma is surely heightened for those taking psychiatric medications:

> I appreciate what medication has done for me, and I recognize that medications like Zoloft, with all its issues, and Wellbutrin, the miracle drug, have improved my life a thousand times over—I don't know where I'd be without them. . . . Would I be a completely different person? And will I ever know that? And can I ever say, "This is who I am" as long as I'm on these? That's my issue with drugs. (female drama student, aged 19)

It is not possible, as Kundera points out, to live two lives to determine the true impact of a single factor (medication vs. no medication, or even illness vs. no illness) on one's self. There are always intervening circumstances—for instance, changing careers, love relationships, or exercise regimens—that may have as much to do with our moods and outlooks as medication does. For the people in my study, this unclear distinction between cause and effect resulted in a great deal of confusion:

And I did get better. Now, was it the Neurontin? Was it the fish oil? Was it the cognitive behavior program which I did for two weeks? What was it? Was it the fact that somebody was paying attention? Was it the fact that I took action and went into the hospital? So what was it? (female writer, aged 59)

And one of the mysteries about it for me is [that] it's hard to know . . . the cause [of my recent pessimism]. Is it the condition itself? Is it the medication? I've been trying cognitive therapy, but it's hard to know how to deal with it when you don't have the facts and you don't know where the problem lies. (male professor, aged 59)

People ask themselves, "If I experience X, is it because of the illness, the medication, or is it 'just me'?" Such confusion not only undercuts the ability to manage one's own illness, as expressed above, but also raises questions about personal identity. The inability to trace with any certainty the causal relationships between one's life experiences, one's illness, and one's drug regimen renders obscure the nature of the authentic self that most of us believe we possess:

Lots of times I haven't had any sense of what's normal for me. Because it's up or down, up or down, and many times in my life I'll say, "What's the real me?

What am I really without the illness?" (female counselor, aged 59)

What if I was really like that [out of control], and I
said I had an illness and I really didn't? I think there
was this huge fear: What if I am this really awful, terrible person but I [just] say I have this illness? (female
sociology student, aged 20)

I don't know whether [my insomnia] is me or
whether it's the medicine. . . . Before I took any medication, I went three years of being an insomniac. So
now, when I stop taking the medicine, I don't know if
it's the fact I stopped taking the medicine, or if it's
just who I am. [Maybe] I'm not meant to sleep. . . . I
don't know any longer [who I am], it's been so long
that I've taken medication, I don't know. (female accountant, aged 29)

There is a subtle but profound sense of loss associated
with such uncertainty. The longing to know the "real me"
is often so powerful that it leads many people to experiment with their medication, sometimes without the
knowledge of their doctors—from trying new drugs or
new combinations of drugs to lowering doses or stopping
medication altogether—in the hopes of determining who
they really are. In a few cases, experimenting with medication did help people clear up some of the confusion created by their illness. For instance, one man, who had been
having serious marital trouble during a deep depression,

thought his illness might have been causing his relationship problems until he removed the depression as a variable:

> It's [trying Prozac] made me realize that . . . my marriage isn't in bad shape because I'm depressed. [It's] in bad shape because we've got shit. . . . The evidence is clear that [after] Prozac . . . my wife and I are [not] . . . being goo-goo, gaa-gaa, and fighting less. (male physician, aged 54)

Going on medication gave this man an opportunity to test a hypothesis about the source of his marital discord. Once he saw that Prozac improved his depression but not his marriage, he had to revise the explanation for his domestic unhappiness.

Many of the people I interviewed experimented by manipulating their dosages of antidepressants. In explaining their motivation for doing so, they spoke of wanting to "go it alone," of experimenting to see if they could handle their problems "on their own." Several described ongoing struggles to reduce the amount of medication they were taking, frequently expressing their ultimate desire to become medication-free. As one male education student, aged twenty, put it: "I mean, I'm kind of working the path to not taking it [Zoloft]. I mean, I'm taking less dosages. . . . I'd like to think, eventually, a year or two maybe, I'll be off the drug completely."

For many, dosage levels were a meaningful indicator of the severity of their illness or, conversely, the degree of

their normalcy. Echoing the observations of several respondents, one man explained, "The goal [is] to keep the
dosages as low as possible . . . [because] it would be nice to
just be a normal person and not have to think about the
medications and so forth." This man and many others
equated less medication with greater authenticity, as if
the lower the dosage the more clearly they could claim
their feelings, thoughts, and actions as their own rather
than as effects of the drugs. As one woman put it, "I wondered if I could sleep without this stuff—and I did it! . . . I
was two pills away from being me." Such sentiments im-
ply a shared belief in the existence of a real self that medications obscure, making a drug-free life the desirable if
elusive goal for many.

The way individuals interpret the relationship between
medications and authenticity affects their attitude toward drug treatments. If, for instance, someone views her
ill self as "the real me," it is not surprising that she would
view medication as an undesirable detour from her "true"
path, however much it may make her feel better. One
woman described her drug treatment as "a deal with the
devil" that she one day hoped to be free of:

> My goal is to not be on medication. I don't want to
> be on meds. I know how helpful they are, and I know
> that they help me and can improve my life. . . . I think
> of the manic-depressive people—the famous ones . . .
> whose talent comes from the fact that they have
> learned how to harness that disability, and I want to
> be able to do the same. . . . I don't want to ignore it or

make it go away, because it's there. Even when I'm on
medication, it's still there, it's just being dealt with
because of the pill. I'd much rather learn to deal with
it . . . because it's a part of me. Depression is a huge
part of my life. . . . [It taught me] to be able to read
myself really well in order to function. So now . . . I
can read a situation really well, and it's one of those
things I pride myself on. . . . And I don't want to lose
that skill. . . . It's something that developed because
of my depression. . . . I want to explore it for a
while. . . . I've decided that I really want to make theater something big in my life. If I can turn depression
into something I can use on stage or as a director
that would be a skill. (female drama student, aged 19)

Like several other interviewees, this woman understood
her depression not only as an undeniable part of who she
was, but also as a teacher, offering valuable skills (and, in
her case, even a career) that carried more meaning than
the improved moods achieved by medication.

Others interpreted the relationship between medication and authenticity differently. Several respondents expressed the belief that their medications did not mask
but rather enabled their true selves, as conveyed by the
remarks of a thirty-year-old man who said, after several
years of taking Zoloft, "It's incredible to discover who I
really am." For this man and others, psychotropic drugs
were the means to recovering a lost self, thus making the
thought of returning to a life before medication unappealing:

I think it was a huge turning point when I wanted to make things better for myself and I wanted to become authentic in the most true sense that I could become authentic. Instead of thinking I was becoming inauthentic by taking medication, I realized that I was totally inauthentic when I wasn't taking medication because I was doing things that made me somebody that I didn't want to be. So it was this sort of paradox in terms of realizing that the medication stood for something positive instead of negative. It took me a while to get there and it wasn't easy, but I got there. (female sociology student, aged 20)

Some individuals may be reluctant to tinker with their drug regimens because they don't want to mess with what works. Several people shared the view expressed by one man who said that "whether it's the real me or not, this is the me that I like." In other words, they so value the ability to function at a high level that they are willing to live with the suspicion that the drugs might somehow distance them from their authentic selves. In addition, some adapt their interpretations of self to fit the ambiguities of their circumstances. A teenager, for example, described coming to the conclusion that she possessed multiple selves, thus effectively safeguarding her sense of authenticity:

I don't have the fears I did anymore . . . that they [medications] would change me. I mean . . . it's kind of like there's two me's. There's the depressed me and there's the happy me. So the depressed me is me, but the nondepressed me is also me. So it's not really changing me. It's just like flipping me over.

It's just making you into one of the me's more often?

Yes, exactly. And I still have a lot of the same views that I had before, but there's a lot less crying and being angry than there was. And it's a whole lot [more fun] being happy. (female high school student, aged 16)

In this chapter we have heard different accounts of the ways psychotropic drugs affect users' senses of themselves. In some cases medication allowed people to realize their authentic selves or to function at a higher level. In this sense their narratives are success stories, even miracles. In other cases, by contrast, people described psychiatric drugs as masking or even devastating their authentic selves. As a result they were typically resistant to or ambivalent about medication.

Although it is impossible to sort out the precise connections among genuine selves, theories of self, and unique life experiences, my interviewees searched within themselves to reclaim or restore lost feelings caused by illness or by medications. Despite different attitudes and life experiences, they shared the common goal of realizing a valued, authentic identity. This search for self is shared by all of us as we repeatedly test, confirm, and revise who we are through experience and experimentation.

Our sense of who we are and how we feel about ourselves is influenced by our communication with others, especially those who are emotionally important in our lives. In a way we are never alone because we carry around in our minds the opinions and expectations of others, a chorus of voices that shape our internal conversations about who we are, what we ought to feel, and how we should act. In the next chapter we will hear how family members, doctors, intimates, and friends influence decisions about taking drugs, the meanings assigned to them, and, ultimately, whether or not they "work."

Chapter 5

Significant Others

In order to embrace . . . medications you have to be open to accepting outside perspectives. I mean, there's something about the medication that is pulling in a whole outside perspective. It's not just taking a pill. It's taking a pill that represents a whole bunch of things. It represents what society thinks about, and what someone else thinks you should do, and what someone else thinks you have.

—female sociology student,

aged 20

Pill-taking is a social act. My conversations about medications contain countless references to significant others— what a parent feels about one's illness, how taking medication affects a spouse, when to tell a new lover about medication use, which friends to confide in, whether to open up to coworkers, and, of course, how caregivers respond to one's feelings and concerns. The meanings people attach to their use of psychotropic drugs are intimately connected with how others view mental illness. Some of the people I talked to bitterly complained that those closest to them simply did not "get it." There are few things more debilitating than sharing your personal story of depression in the hope of feeling less alone, only to have people question your perspectives, your decisions in dealing with the problem, or even the problem's very existence.[1] Many people feel pressured by loved ones to take medications they do not want to take or to stop taking medications they believe are necessary for their well-being. Several of these themes are present in Alison's story.

Alison was the first person I interviewed for this book. At the time we spoke she was a college junior struggling to maintain a high grade point average while battling depression. As with many others, her struggle was compounded by the fear of how important people in her life would react to her illness. It was, for example, no easy thing for this young woman to tell her boyfriend that she was suffering from a mental illness severe enough to require medication. Although he turned out to be a mainstay in her life, Alison said: "It took me six months of therapy and a support group to be able to tell my boyfriend [I was taking medications]. I was with him for a year before I told him." When I asked her to elaborate she told me:

> My biggest fear in life is that people are going to find out and they're going to run in the other direction. And that I'm going to be alone and I'm going to spend the rest of my life alone. It's been a huge, huge fear. And a burden. Such a burden. So that's one of

the reasons I think people at some point on drugs
want to stop taking them. In the long run who wants
to be with someone who's mentally ill? . . . Who
wants to spend the rest of their life with someone
who is going to be depressed and who is going to be
like always taking medicine and always have this part
of them that's just not . . . happy and good?

Alison's fears about losing important people in her life
who either could not understand the severity of her depression or were afraid to maintain ties with someone ill
enough to sometimes contemplate suicide were not un-
founded. She told me: "Last year, a girl who I've known
since my freshman year in college, who I consider my closest friend at school, I told about my depression and, you
know, the medication and everything. And I got a bad response from her." Fearing the loss of still other friends,
Alison decided to remain largely silent about her illness.
There is, though, a substantial price to pay for this strategy: the paradox of silence is that while it may shield sufferers from the disapproval of others, it can lead to isolation. Rather than feigning wellness, people often retreat
from social circles. Alison captured the tension between
remaining isolated and being inauthentic:

I am alone because sympathy is one thing, but empathy is another and people just don't get it. And they
can be sympathetic, but I don't tell anyone. I mean, I
definitely don't ever say, "Hey, I'm going off my medicine." I now have a few friends who I tell who know

that I'm depressive and that I take medication, but
when I'm switching from one to the other or when
something's going on, I don't tell anyone.

A colleague of mine once described therapists as "paid
friends." Most patients and therapists would likely balk
at such a description, claiming that friendship has no
place in the client-therapist relationship, that, in fact, the
development of a friendship between patient and healer
would actually undermine the therapeutic relationship.[2]
At the same time, when asked about what they want from
a therapist, most people describe a relationship similar to
an intimate friendship. In Alison's case, her doctor continued to see her even though she did not have the money
to pay him. She said: "I've been extremely fortunate with
my psychopharmacologist. In two years he has received
three hundred and twenty-five dollars. He sees me every
other week because I haven't found the right medication
in two years. He is constantly there for me." When asked
what made him such a good doctor, she explained that he
is "someone who listens to your concerns and hears you
clearly before taking out the prescription pad and writing
down a medicine. . . . He really listens to me and to what I
want." Like a good friend, her doctor made a concerted
effort to hear and understand her story.

Shortly before our conversation Alison had taken a
part-time job with the intention of paying her doctor in
full. Indeed, the matter of money led us to the most compelling part of her medication story. She was struggling
to honor her medical bills because of her parents' deci-

sion to stop paying for her treatment. Her "antipill family" had come to the conclusion that Alison should not be taking psychiatric medications. Alison felt thoroughly misunderstood by her parents and a sister who believed that she was exaggerating her suffering and that, if anything, her illness was caused by the medications she was taking. They had even consulted a relative who was a physician in a distant state and had never talked with Alison about her emotional difficulties. Neither distance nor lack of knowledge about Alison's situation prevented him from supporting the family's antipill bias. Here's how Alison described the pressure she felt to stop taking medication:

> It goes back to my mother and my father. My mom . . . has never been there for me and has never accepted my depression. She thinks that since I've had such a hard time taking medicine—you know, been through so many—that I should just go to herbal remedies now and just forget about it. My sister thinks that I should . . . do acupuncture . . . because my medicine is not working. The link is that they don't think that I should be on medication. They think I'm wasting money and wasting time. My mom's theory is that if I stopped thinking about it so much, I would be fine. And I should just not go to therapy and not see any doctors and just not think about it. And my response is that if I don't think about it and I don't take care of it, then I'm not going to be alive. My dad's theory is that I take too

much medicine and that I took medicine too early
and that's what is wrong with me now. [He thinks]
that the medicine messed me up. . . . And my sister's
theory is that she's doing fine without medication
[so] I could be doing fine without medication.

Alison concluded by saying:

It makes it difficult to take medicine.

It is no wonder that in the face of such opposition
Alison stopped taking medication from time to time.
That she persevered in obtaining the treatment she believed she needed was in fact testament to her personal
strength. After all, in numerous studies social psychologists have shown the power of groups in getting people to
conform to their demands.[3] I imagine that nearly every
reader of this book can think of situations in their lives
when they gave in to family pressure.

Alison's dilemma surrounding medication use high-
lights the role of family, therapists, intimate others, and
friends in shaping the way we view drug therapy. In the
remainder of this chapter I will explore the influence of
each of these categories of significant others in shaping
the meanings given to medications.

Family

What we learn in the context of our families carries great
emotional significance and typically shapes our attitudes,

values, and perspectives for a lifetime. Much has been written about the influence of childhood socialization on such matters as gender, race, and ethnic and religious ideas. However, childhood lessons about the body, illness, and pain are also among the most enduring. Comparative investigations of illness show that the meanings attached to physical and mental symptoms vary from society to society, that decisions about what constitutes disease are as much social products as they are purely medical ones.[4] In much the same way, definitions of illnesses and what to do about them vary among ethnic, racial, class, religious, and family groups within the same society. For example, researchers have repeatedly demonstrated ethnic differences in the experiences and meanings attached to pain.[5] We should not be surprised to learn, therefore, that people's attitudes toward medications for emotional pain cannot be separated from their parents' attitudes about pain and pills. One woman described the ease with which she took psychiatric drugs after having grown up in a family where pills were pervasive:

> My father and my mother [took lots of pills]. In our spice rack, and this is what I grew up with, in our spice rack . . . we didn't have spices. We had pills and we had pills for going to sleep, for waking up, [and] amphetamines to get through the day. My father had many medical illnesses, so he was on a lot of meds. And my mother felt that for every problem you had there was a medication to take. So that's kind of how I learned. (female health advocate, aged 57)

One man with a long family history of mental illness found beginning drug therapy unproblematic:

> My mother is manic-depressive and I had seen her being resistant to taking drugs, and she would go off her lithium because she wanted to escape her marital problems, and her way of doing it was to go off of her medication and get hospitalized so she didn't have to stay in the house. . . . So I learned from watching what she was doing that these kind of people need to stay on their lithium. . . . My family is definitely pro-meds. (retail salesman, aged 36)

As the short version of Alison's story illustrated, the decision to embark on a course of medication and to stick with it is far more difficult when family members, parents in particular, are skeptical about treating emotional pain with medications. One of the most difficult things for people suffering from the debilitating pain of depression and anxiety is to have family members discount their complaints or to invalidate their illness experiences altogether.

Several people I interviewed had grown up in households where complaining about emotional problems was seen as whining. Parents who believed in the ethic of toughing it out and solving one's own problems usually disapproved of a son's or daughter's decision to use medication. This disapproval contributed to patients' pain by making them feel misunderstood at a moment when they needed others to believe their story and react with compassion. Affective disorders are illnesses of isolation. The isolation is greatly magnified when family members minimize the pain and one's approach to dealing with it:

I would curl up in the bathroom, in my room, just crying uncontrollably, not knowing what was wrong with me, and at the same time being very irritable because no one was very sensitive to it. . . . My mom was actually starting to go on medication for depression at the same time, and I think she had a bad experience with therapists, not feeling that they were worth anything. And so I said to her, "You know, I really need to talk to someone," and she told me, "Well, you should just keep a journal about how you feel . . . because that's what they'll ask you to do if you see somebody." And that was kind of the end of it, and I just kind of gave up after that, because I felt like, "Man, if I keep a journal it's going to be too late. That's just ridiculous." (male sociology student, aged 22)

I just got pissed at them [parents]. . . . They sort of said that they thought that the drugs were the cause of my recent . . . downfall and that they'd tried to read up on some of them. And I guess they talked to my brother, this physician, and he didn't know shit about drugs. And they thought that I should just get off them because it's causing me problems. (female homemaker, aged 28)

I pleaded and begged with my mother to try to understand. . . . She claims she understood the best that she could, but I just . . .

Why was it important for you to have your mother understand?

Well, this is my mother, number one, and I'm under the same roof with her. I love her and I wanted her support and understanding of what I was going through . . . from the withdrawal [from medications]. And I said the best thing you can do is understand and to educate yourself. . . . I wanted my mother there. I wanted her compassion. I wanted her understanding. I wanted her to be there. And she just . . . she doesn't get it. So I've given up with that with her. (female market researcher, aged 35)

The power of parental expectations can be seen in the case of a doctor who repeatedly mentioned the necessity of taking his medications. As a physician, he understood the biological mechanisms through which pills affect the human body. As someone with personal experience of depression, he could also describe the pills as lifesavers. Yet with all his knowledge, both medical and personal, he found it hard to put aside his parents' antimedication perspective, and even stopped medications on occasion to please them:

> My mother was the type that would, if I said I had a headache, she'd say, "You're a whiny kid." There was no caring if you were ill, there was no tenderness. In fact, you were supposed to be a good little soldier. My parents . . . are staunchly antimedication. I remember on many occasions my father saying, "The slightest thing that goes wrong with you and all you want to do is take another pill." And so when I was starting to do well, I wanted to be able to please my parents by being able to come off the medications.

The dilemmas posed by parental expectations cut in two directions. In many instances interviewees described situations where family members coerced them into taking medications they wanted to avoid. Such pressure is, of course, most successfully applied to children. In Chapter 6 I will explore the particular difficulties faced by children who have been told they must take medications. We should not be surprised, however, that young people sometimes feel great distress and anger at having pills "shoved down their throats." One woman remembered battling with her mother, a therapist, who refused to respect her wishes to avoid medication:

> She was for it. She pushed medication—pushed it, pushed it, pushed it. She's always, "You need medica-

tion. You need medication." So she thought it was terrific I was on it. . . . I have some anger toward her because she pushed the goddamn medications. . . . She thought it would help me. I wouldn't be so depressed. . . . My mother has heard me scream at her many a time, "Stop fucking analyzing me and keep your job at the office." (female graduate student, aged 29)

When I went off [medications], I would get violent. My mother would immediately say, "See, this is what happens. This is because you're depressed." I was saying, "No [it's from withdrawal]." I was staying on this medication, and the more I stayed on it the more I resented it. . . . I was getting [from her], "This is a return of your depression." My mother was great at diagnosing me. But as far as keeping me on medication, I really resent her in a lot of areas. I would say, "I have to work through it. I have to learn to live without medication because I don't want to depend on a pill for the rest of my life." (female drama student, aged 19)

Several people recalled that medication had become a power struggle in which they would subvert their parents' demands:

I lied a lot about taking it. My mom used to fill one of those pill boxes, and I was supposed to take it.

What ended up happening a lot is that I would take it a couple of days. And then the weekend would come and I wouldn't take it over the weekend. . . . But my mom always gave them to me. For a long time I wasn't allowed to have the pills. She had to bring them to me at night. . . . It was very much a power struggle between Mom and Dad and me. They would come in and [say], "There's your pills." And I don't want them. . . . I used to torture my mother. . . . I would engage her in these power struggles. Well, they would ask if I had taken my pills. And I would say yes. And a lot of the time I knew they would find out that I hadn't. And again they had to come confront me about that. (female sociology student, aged 20)

I was forgetting so much [that] my mom thought, "Well, maybe a pill case will help you because you can see the days and see when you take it and when you didn't take it," and I was like, "Oh, so now I'm like an old person. I have all these pills." That was definitely like a power struggle. It was a power struggle because I was like, "No, I'm a kid, I don't need a pill case." But she was like, "You obviously need it because you're not remembering." So there was a time when I was . . . "Eh, pill case." (female education student, aged 19)

This section has emphasized some of the confusion and negative emotions that can result when families disagree about the appropriateness of drug therapies for emotional problems. But I also heard from people whose families seemed to "get it" and to offer unqualified support. One woman described "a sister who was very supportive when I first went to the hospital. She wrote me a poem about lithium . . . that she loved me whether I was on lithium or not. It was lovely." Another spoke of a brother who "was on lithium . . . and so he was a great source of help for me." Yet another woman supported her sister's drug therapy, saying, "It's so wonderful. I feel like I finally got my sister back again after twenty years." Several others described "incredibly supportive families."

As much as family attitudes toward drug treatment arouse strong emotions and shape medication decisions, the strongest feelings expressed by interviewees were reserved for therapists. Typically, the people interviewed for this study had dealt with several categories of mental health professionals over the years—family doctors, talk therapists, psychiatrists, and psychopharmacologists. Virtually everyone had had both positive and negative experiences with care providers. All had strong and remarkably similar ideas about what distinguishes good and bad doctors. Not surprisingly, their criteria centered on the capacity or willingness of those who treated them to truly hear, understand, and respect their illness accounts. Equally, those who had experimented with medications over years, sometimes decades, had developed expertise about medications that they believed warranted a more egalitarian doctor-patient relationship than current professional models normally allow.

Therapy

There is an old joke that begins with the observation that among those who invest time and money in talk therapy about one-third get better, one-third stay the same, and one-third get worse. The punch line is that among emotionally troubled people who avoid any sort of talk therapy about one-third get better, one-third stay the same, and one-third get worse. Jokes aside, there is evidence that many people find talk therapy helpful.[6] While it is difficult to evaluate the effectiveness of therapy scientifically, we cannot quarrel with individuals' self-reports on the value of therapy for enhancing their well-being. More provocative are studies suggesting that nearly *all* forms of psychotherapy are effective.[7] According to the psychiatrist Arthur Kleinman, for example, both mainstream, medically sanctioned therapies and less conventional therapies can be equally successful. At the root of healing is not the extent of the therapist's training but the patient's belief in the therapist and the particular symbolic system on which the therapy is based:

> What is necessary for healing to occur is that both
> parties to the therapeutic transaction are committed
> to the shared symbolic order. What is important is
> that the patient has the opportunity to tell his story,
> experiences the therapist's witnessing of the account,
> believes the therapist's interpretation of his prob-
> lems, and comes to use the same symbolic vehicles of

> interpretation to make sense of his situation. Because of his own need to believe and the rhetorical skills of the therapist to make key symbols relevant to the experience of the sufferer, the sick person becomes convinced that a transformation of his experience is possible and is in fact happening.[8]

While it makes sense that a patient's relationship with a healer would substantially affect the outcome of talk therapy, we might assume that any placebo effect is less powerful when it comes to medications that presumably work by changing levels of neurotransmitters in people's brains. Yet here again drug trials demonstrate that placebo effects "vary between 10 and 90 percent . . . and seem to be strongly influenced by the quality of the doctor-patient relationship."[9] Given its powerful effects, it is odd that medicine largely considers the placebo effect a nuisance factor in determining the independent effects of the drugs themselves. As drug companies, researchers, teachers, and psychiatrists become committed to the view that people with affective disorders suffer from broken brains, purely and simply, the quality of doctor-patient relations becomes a peripheral concern: "Biomedicine is the major system of healing in the West. Yet it has little to do with what is most central to most healing systems, symbolic healing."[10]

During the conversations I had for this book nearly every person had stories to tell about good and bad doctors. Implicit in their remarks was the notion that the quality of their relationships with mental health professionals matters greatly; there was more to it than merely leaving their offices with a prescription for medications. Julie, a twenty-nine-year-old graduate student in English litera-ture, explicitly tied her wellness and the success of her medications to her relationships with doctors. She ex-plained: "[The medications work] because I believe the person, and the people, myself included, coming up with the ideas about which drugs might be best [for me] have my best interest at heart. And they take time with me and listen and don't always just brush things away."

Julie continued by describing an unfortunate incident. She and her regular psychiatrist made a joint decision to seek a consultation with a well-known psychopharma-cologist who, unlike her psychiatrist, was an "expert" on bipolar illness. Her psychiatrist prepared "a three- to five-paged single-spaced very good description of everything [that had happened] over the past five years." When she arrived for the appointment, it became immediately clear that the new doctor had not bothered to read the report, nor could he find it when asked. Outraged that she had spent a very expensive hour recapitulating her case, Julie later left a phone message complaining to the consultant about his lack of preparation: "He called me back and on my [answering] machine and said, 'I got your message. There will be no appointment next week. . . . You clearly have issues. There will be no appointment.'" She finished her account with these observations:

> His power was threatened by this little dumb girl who
> just came along, who's crazy, and when he got threat-

ened he said, "I'm going to throw her out before she throws me out." And that's what he did. . . . I literally believe that he would only play out the . . . role of power doctor, megaman, young and upcoming star. And when little old me, this poor little stupid graduate student [showed up] . . . he just knew I looked young. I was a woman, probably a girl in his mind. When I tried to break his picture of his own performance as this high-powered guy, he couldn't deal [with it]. . . . He couldn't even allow for the possibility of fracturing his performative image. And it would only work if I came in, you know, sort of self-loathing and weak and saying, "Help me." And self-deprecating, and "You're the master, I'll do whatever you say." . . . I think . . . that everything is so [socially] constructed that even the biological effect of a single pill on the same person and the same dosage taken at the same time every day could be completely different depending upon who's prescribing it.

Earlier in this chapter I talked about the important role of families in childhood socialization. However, socialization continues throughout our lives. In our jobs, our role as spouses, parents, and eventually new retirees, we must learn how to function. Learning how to deal with illness, doctors, and medications also involves a steep learning curve. At the outset of an illness, patients often feel helpless and unquestioningly give themselves over to the care of doctors. Despite the proliferation of information available on the Internet and in drug advertising aimed directly at the public, new patients often have difficulty expressing clear opinions about drug treatment. During the early stages of illness careers, typically characterized by desperation and vulnerability, patients largely follow doctors' orders. In retrospect, many of those in my sample eventually came to feel that their doctors had not initially provided them with enough information about their illness:

> I wasn't savvy. I didn't know how to go about choosing the right person. I didn't know where to go. I mean, I felt that it was me. Part of this whole process is if I didn't get better, it was my fault. It didn't have anything to do with a clinician's fault. It was my fault. It was deserved. It was me. (male media consultant, aged 52)

> If she had only said to me, "Listen, Klonopin is addictive and there are side effects, withdrawal," or just anything. At least I would have had the choice whether to take it or not. But she didn't say any of that. So I just assumed and listened to her. I mean, I'm just trusting this doctor and I took it. And if she had just said that word "dependent" or "addictive," that would have been it for me. I would have never taken one. That's what gets me angry because then I could have decided whether or not I wanted to take it. (female market researcher, aged 35)

With psychiatry's embrace of a purely biomedical model of mental illness, doctors have increasingly failed to meet patients' needs for empathy and intimacy. In the end, though, the biggest disappointment for patients may be the realization that doctors cannot easily fix them. Depressed and anxious people are likely to have strong expectations that physicians will solve their problems. After all, TV spots lament the fact that so few people with depression are diagnosed since it is such a treatable disease. Drug companies routinely quote a success rate of 80 percent for their products. However, as earlier chapters suggest, stories of complete success are far less common than stories of mixed results or resistance to treatment. At some point in the patient socialization process, most people must come to terms with the fact that their illness is not going away.

When initial expectations for a quick solution fade and patients find themselves on the roller coaster of hope and disillusionment, their view of medical expertise and the role that they must play in their own recovery become more balanced. As I will show in the Epilogue, the people I spoke with shared the belief that patients must become knowledgeable consumers by researching the drugs they take, by carefully shopping for doctors, and by generally adopting a more activist role in their own care. Many of those I interviewed came to trust their own experience and knowledge over the presumed expertise of their doctors. Comments like "there's a subtle understanding that can only come from the inside"; or "I'd feel better if the doctors were taking the pills [too]," assert the validity of personal knowledge and a growing faith in one's own expertise. Such a cognitive shift typically generates displeasure with the hierarchical structure of doctor-patient relationships:

> Well, I have a theory about our relationship with psychiatrists. I am convinced that those of us who have depression or manic depression must be in charge of our medical doings. . . . We have to have enough trust in the doctor or doctors that we're dealing with. And they have to have enough trust in us to let us be in charge. They may not always agree with us, and sometimes they have to take chances. (retired small business owner, aged 68)

> And I kept on saying to my doctor, "Would you consider prescribing this medication?" I had heard this medication had worked dramatically for people who have had these refractory conditions. And she said, "Well, I don't know enough about it." I said, "Well, can you call this doctor who does prescribe it liberally?" She really didn't do it. Finally, in one session, and there were a number of sessions where I was just tearful because nothing was happening, and I just felt that I was just losing [my] grip. And I said, "Let me ask you something. If you were me, what would you do?" And she shifted uncomfortably in her chair and said, "I'd be a cowboy." I left with that script that day. A cowboy means they are willing to take risks. And it's because of that question, that one question, that

use of that language in a way to say, "Put yourself in
my place, forget about the vertical relationship that
normally exists between you and me and let's just
switch gears here." And it was just amazing. (male
media consultant, aged 52)

Sometimes I don't think they take it seriously
enough. Like it's very easy for them to pull out a prescription pad and switch things around or add something new. . . . Maybe they see twenty patients a day
and are managing their medications, and maybe
they're not always looking at it from your perspective.
(female research assistant, aged 22)

Sometimes, disenchantment with a doctor's expertise
leads a patient to even more strident demands for equal-
ity in decision-making processes:

And I sometimes feel . . . that they think we're stupid.
I feel like we're little guinea pigs. Try this. And try
that drug. I was taking Risperdal or something like
that. And I said, "I don't like how I felt." So I took it
for two nights and so I stopped taking it. And he
said, "Well, you should have called me." And I was
like, "I don't have to do anything. I shouldn't have to
call you. It didn't work. I didn't like the way it made
me feel. That's enough. Thanks. And I'm here, aren't
I?" And in that respect, I just feel that they think we
owe them something. But I don't even think about
that anymore. And I realize it's my time [with the

doctor] and I can do whatever I want to with it. It's back to compliance. I don't have to comply with what they expect of me. I'm paying them money, so they're going to listen to what I have to say. (female sociology student, aged 20)

My interviewees expressed the least animosity toward traditional psychotherapists, whose approach, after all, centers on stories.[11] In contrast, the greatest criticism was reserved for psychiatrists who listened only to reports of symptoms and whose central tool was the prescription pad: "They don't want to deal with people's issues"; "He's not trying for one second to think about what it's like to be in the other person's shoes"; "He didn't seem to care or understand."

Patients were most satisfied with doctors who recommended a combination of psychotherapy and drug treatment and considered this to be a natural division of labor between professionals. Although most of the people I interviewed expressed dissatisfaction with doctors who were exclusively pill oriented, others described the deep and mutual trust that can develop with psychopharmacologists:

They watch you get through really tough times and they develop some respect for you. And they prescribe some things that actually make a difference and you develop some respect for them. And as that happens, trust develops and you are willing to try things that

you weren't willing to try and weather storms that
might get worse. (unemployed woman, aged 47)

The biomedical model of illness makes patients' stories increasingly irrelevant to treatment.[12] Medical students are socialized to view their expertise in terms of proper diagnosis and treatment. Moreover, as medicine becomes ever more specialized, the patient in room 303 becomes the gallbladder or the type II bipolar. The depersonalization of patients and the increasing lack of interest in their stories are accelerated by insurance companies that place their premiums exclusively on diagnostic categories. As health care costs escalate, doctors face increasing caseloads, specific rules about how much time they can spend with each patient, and a mountain of paperwork. Taken together, these circumstances lead doctors to complain justifiably that they "never have enough time."[13] Unfortunately, the vital truth that "hearing heals" becomes largely lost in such a professional context.

Intimacy

Sometimes people are so intent on establishing intimate ties that they systematically present attitudes, values, behaviors, and self-images that they believe will be acceptable to others. They carefully choose the information they share in order to make a good first impression. During courtship, in particular, each person typically offers an idealized self-image and is willing to accept the idealized image the other presents. For someone with a history of emotional illness and psychiatric drug use, new relationships pose complicated dilemmas: Should I tell? When is the right time? How should I do it? One young man described his strategy:

> Initially, when I meet someone, yeah, I'm thinking, "Okay, at what point do I tell them that I have this side of my life?" You know, new women that I meet. Part of it is you don't want them to think about that [medications] when they think about you. You don't want that to be a part of your identity when, in fact, it is a part of your identity. It's kind of the dark secret in the closet. . . . When it comes to depression, I'll say, "Yeah, I take this medication." Sometimes, if we're drinking, I'll say, "Oh, I can't drink too much." They'll say, "Why?" I'll say, "Oh, because I take this medication." "Oh, what's the medication?" "It's Celexa. It's an antidepressant." I kind of lead it in that way. I don't just come out and say, "I have depression." [I'm] kind of trying interesting ways to get around it to where I make it sound as if it's not a big deal. (male peace activist, aged 22)

As relationships deepen and appear to have long-term potential, questions of disclosure become more pressing. Two interviewees talked specifically about the need to consider their medicine cabinets once it became clear that a potential partner might be spending time in their apartments. The similarity of their comments is striking:

I've always been fascinated by why people go off medications. . . . And you know, there's nothing that screams mental illness to your face any more than opening up that medicine chest. . . . I mean, what if I get into a relationship and, you know, I don't want to tell my girlfriend or something that I have a psychiatric illness or open up the medicine chest? So . . . it's basically telling you every day, every time you take that pill, that you're ill and all the stigma that goes with it. (male physician, aged 44)

When I started new relationships I would get really uncomfortable, especially if he started staying over, or whatever, that there would be these times when I would conceal that I was taking medication. Not that anyone ever thought that I was sick, because, you know, you're on this high from being in a relationship. But I was afraid that I would be found out. . . . I know that I felt a lot of hesitance in continuing in drug therapy when there was a new relationship in my life. . . . I think that's because . . . when there's somebody else in the picture you start thinking about yourself in different ways. [There is] this anticipation of . . . what's going to happen on this day? Are we going to kiss? Is he going to come up? Is he going to spend the night? type of thing. . . . You know, if he starts staying over you've got to go and sort of reconfigure your medicine cabinet, for lack of a better term. . . . You have to think about your presentation of self. (female homemaker, aged 28)

In fact, Andrea, whose words you just read, was in a serious relationship and about to marry at the time we talked. She had recently learned that she was pregnant, and both she and Mark, her partner, were looking forward to a new life together. The pregnancy, however, further complicated Andrea's decision about remaining on medication.[14] Now she had to consider both the potential dangers of her drug regimen for the baby and Mark's view of her. She finally stopped taking the drugs altogether. She described how she reached that decision:

> I had a lot of anxiety going to the obstetrician because they have to ask you all this stuff and I have decisions to make. . . . You know, I wanted Mark to be a part of the process of being there for the visits and asking his own questions. . . . I had my normal anxiety of what person am I going to let him know me as . . . as somebody who has taken drugs a couple of times a day? . . . [Finally,] I stopped taking my medication. I think it was two things . . . being with Mark . . . and compromising the baby. So I just stopped. I didn't want it [medications] to touch this new phase of my life. I just saw it as a shadow of some sort, and I just didn't want it. I didn't want it to be there for this.

Several people found themselves in a difficult double bind. Intimacy demands honesty, yet questions of authenticity do not stop with disclosure of one's psychiatric history. Recall that people suffering from mental illnesses like depression remain deeply confused about whether they are more authentically themselves on or off drugs. The matter can be especially perplexing for those who have remained on medication since their relationship began. Although one partner may know about the other's illness, he may never have seen her during episodes of depression or mania. Consider the dilemma faced by a newlywed whose sexual response was diminished by the SSRI she was taking. She wanted to experience the full intensity of intimacy in her marriage. Yet to stop taking the drug might mean revealing unappealing sides of herself to her new husband:

> I think his preference is that I wouldn't be on the medication. He's really said it to me in so many words. . . . He feels like I can be more of my [sexual] self if I'm not on it. . . . In the time that we've known each other, it has been a positive time for me. And I've been on medication the whole time. He's never seen me in a really dark period. . . . And can I tolerate the [bad] feelings in order to experience the full range of who I am [sexually]? Sometimes, even now, when I start losing my temper, and that's rare, I'm embarrassed by it. I don't want him to see me that way, even though I think he would be really good about it. But it's still hard for me. . . . I don't think there's any clear solution. (female technical writer, aged 50)

Thus far I have been describing how use of psychiatric medications influences the way people present themselves during the *construction* of intimate relationships. As the newlywed's comments suggest, however, decisions about medication influence the *preservation* of intimate relationships as well. After the initial stage of courtship, partners find it increasingly difficult to maintain idealized images of each other. Day-to-day life melts away initial impressions, often revealing attitudes, values, behaviors, and emotional frailties that were previously well guarded. To be sure, among the people I interviewed pills often became the basis for conflict. One woman ended a three-year relationship because "he was very, very much against the whole psychiatric profession [and] didn't believe I had an illness. . . . He thought that I fetishized pills." Another man said: "My wife kind of had trouble with it [medication] after we got married. . . . I actually got to know her when I was much healthier." Someone else explained: "My wife wants me to give it all up. . . . It's a totally uninformed feeling . . . and I keep telling her that if she had my problem she would probably want to be on medication too." In a very different circumstance, going on a "medication holiday" (deciding to take a break from medication for a while) upset an established division of labor between partners:

> During those two months when I wasn't on any medication, I was feeling pretty good and feeling kind of frisky in our relationship. I would say that Beverly is . . . more the doer, the task person. I'm more of a thinker, contemplative. And I think I started to do more things. . . . I think that Beverly was reacting to kind of a new person when I got like that . . . and

> even the way I am now. I mean, she loves to see me
> feeling well, but there are those adjustments that she
> has to make. I mean, she's always been the cook in
> the kitchen and I do the cleaning up. When I'm feel-
> ing good, cooking looks kind of interesting so I . . .
> start puttering around there. And the kitchen is kind
> of Beverly's domain. (female administrative aide,
> aged 54)

Just as suddenly becoming well can pose identity problems for someone who has struggled with depression, the
sudden wellness of an intimate other can undermine a
couple's collective identity. Such a negative wellness effect
is unhappily illustrated in Rita's case. Rita had been in
a long-term committed relationship when she was diagnosed with bipolar disorder. For years she had been oper-
ating in a hypomanic state characterized by dizzying periods of activity and productivity. Like many others, Rita
had gone undiagnosed because she had always been defined as an enormously productive, super-achieving, and
creative professional. The character of her illness did not
become clear until the hypomania became a full-blown
psychotic episode. Once she started taking lithium, Rita's
mania was controlled, but she had become a different person to her partner. Because Rita was unwilling to change
her medication regimen, the relationship fell apart:

> Things have been more complicated with my partner.
> The Rita she fell in love with was the hypomanic Rita,
> and then she ended up with this person who was for

a while very sluggish and whatnot . . . and it wasn't at all healthy for our relationship. And she felt that I shouldn't be on so much medicine—that it would solve everything if I just would ask [my doctor] to decrease my medication. And I wasn't going to do that. I mean, I knew that my levels were appropriate and I needed to be where I was, and I was doing all the things I needed to be doing and there was no way I was going to ask [my doctor] to lower my medication.

She wanted you more revved up?

She wanted me more revved up, and I knew that, and I basically told her on more than one occasion that the hypomanic Rita was never coming back, that she had to just get used to that idea. The long and short of it is that we broke up last September. (female physician, aged 46)

For nearly all those who are uncertain or distressed by their partners' turn to medication, there are those who believe unequivocally that their significant others need medication and encourage them to seek treatment. Mental illness takes a terrible toll on relationships, eroding the bonds of intimacy.[15] Even people in long-term committed relationships find that mental illness challenges the solidity of their lives together. Frank described his marriage as unusually strong and intimate but noted that he overcame his resistance to medication only when his wife made it clear that "I needed to see a shrink and that I needed to be on medication." Frank understood his wife's insistence as evidence that "she's deeply concerned about me. She wanted me to be happier." He remembered one incident in particular when her message finally "got through":

> Once we were on the golf course in the summertime, me and my wife. And I was walking around with a deep face and not being able to enjoy the beautiful day, and she stops, and she said, "Frank, look around you, you see all these people playing? Every one of them has got a problem like you've got, virtually every one of them. But they're here and they're having fun. You need to do something." . . . She's like, "Come on, if there's a pill for it, take it, for God's sake . . . What's the downside? Go on the pills." (male teacher, aged 57)

As noted in Chapter 2, the medical literature on patient compliance with medication is enormous. The assumption underlying much of the discussion is that if only doctors could better communicate to patients the necessity of following a medication regimen, compliance would increase. This may be so. However, medical treatment built on the presumption of a two-person social system—doctor and patient—misses the way each of us is embedded in a network of significant others.[16] As the accounts in this section demonstrate, people's attitudes toward psychotropic drug use are inseparable from the perspectives and concerns of those with whom they wish to build or to sustain an intimate relationship. Along with family members, therapists, and intimate others, friends and colleagues influence how the meanings of psychotropic medications are socially constructed.

Solidarity

While some people remain lifelong friends, most of us move through different circles as the circumstances of our lives change. People who are heading toward marriage typically experience a realignment of friendships—what Peter Berger and Hansfried Kellner have less kindly called the "liquidation" of former friends.[17] When babies arrive, single friends may make way for others who will not be bored with discussions of diaper preferences, first words, or the best places to shop for children's clothes. People in similar stages in their careers often become fast friends. Likewise, illness dramatically reshapes life circumstances, self-conceptions, and the circle of people who can appreciate what one is "going through." Friends often become obsolete when dramatic shifts in experience and identity make it impossible for them to understand one's new world:

> My best friend, who had no idea what was going on
> in my life, didn't feel the things that I felt. No one
> else thought about death all the time. No one else
> thought that they'd rather be dead. They all thought
> it was a bad thing. I thought it was a good thing. . . .
> Really, the only people who mattered to me were my

friends who were depressed like me. (female accountant, aged 29)

My best friend, after I told her that they were going to start me on medication, she just started crying on the telephone. She said, "Oh, but I'm so afraid that it will change your personality." (female research assistant, aged 22)

I did push away a lot of people. Mostly because I felt that they didn't understand. And if I felt that they didn't really understand or were just sort of nodding and trying to be friends but not really getting it, I didn't want to sit there and feel like I was being patronized even though they really did care. It wasn't the same as finding solace in somebody who I felt understood what I was going through. (female homemaker, aged 28)

The people I interviewed said their friendships faded away either because they did not feel understood by their former friends or because their friends withdrew out of fear and lack of understanding:

A lot of friends have been very supportive over the years. But I think it has limited their friendship. [They're] not willing to get involved in things they can't cope with. Yeah, you get a reassortment of friends. (female writer, aged 58)

You get very isolated. Your friends stop calling. My friends are calling again, but they weren't calling for a while. When the medication was starting to work they started calling again, but when I had severe symptoms, they were saying things like, "My husband and my daughter are my priority." And they were kind of like, "Take a walk." . . . I mean, people that were friends for twenty-five years were saying this to me. So it was really awful, and other people have just gone out of my life. (unemployed woman, aged 47)

Over and again the message is the same. People need empathy and understanding. The anguish of mental illness is heightened when family members, therapists, partners, and friends do not comprehend one's suffering. Indeed, the pain of depression arises in part from an inability to connect even as one yearns for such connection. Depressed people typically isolate themselves because "when you are alone and depressed you don't feel that you have to be something that you're not for other people." Such isolation is, however, a kind of false economy, since being alone with the experience eventually deepens the depression.

Having spent many years as a member of a support group for depression and manic depression, I appreciate the almost magical power that comes from the simple feeling that others know your plight. The power of such support groups also comes from the liberation that follows being able to remove false masks. Every week at the meetings of the Manic-Depressive and Depressive Association people talk freely about difficult life problems, including periods of hospitalization and years of drug therapy. To drop the cloak of secrecy about a stigmatized condition is liberating and healing. Tom, one of the people I recruited for this study at MDDA, explained why his closest friends now come from that group:

> My friends are people who go to MDDA. I've met
> them there. I've gotten to know them there, and a lot
> of the barriers of personal information are down
> there, and it makes it a lot easier to get to know
> somebody. . . . You don't have to worry about a lot of
> the social [things]. . . . Well, the stigma's not there.
> You don't have to worry about whether or not you're
> going to disclose that you have a disability to people.
> It's just a lot easier. (retail salesman, aged 36)

Tom's comments about stigma and disclosure echo many of the conversations throughout this book. Like those suffering from a wide variety of physical illnesses, people with emotional issues must also decide whether to disclose their psychiatric problems at work. Discussion at MDDA meetings often centered on these questions: How might individuals explain significant gaps in their work histories? Should someone admit to prior hospitalizations? What should be said to interviewers who ask if anything might compromise their job performance? Once on the job, should one tell supervisors and coworkers about an illness that can be incapacitating from time to time? Can coworkers become confidants? Repeated stories of workplace discrimination toward people with psychiatric illnesses normally led to a simple and shared conclusion: "Don't tell!" For most, then, work became another life domain requiring secrecy and the additional burdens it brought:

> I wouldn't tell anyone at work. I'm still into that work-secrecy thing. (male physician, aged 54)

> I didn't [normally] think about it during the day. But every time the medication came out, which . . . would be like three or four times a day, I was just constantly being reminded of it. Every time you pull out those medications, it's a reminder of that. And I mean, I was working in a little cubicle, but it's like I have to hide. . . . I mean, people take medication there, but I felt like I had to hide it. (female psychology student, aged 21)

One of the most surprising things I have learned from conversations with doctors is that of all occupations, medicine seems to be the least forgiving of illnesses, especially mental illnesses. I first sensed this when a family friend, a physician who had just read my earlier book on depression, called me at home. He was eager to talk about the book and about his struggles with depression. When he said that this was one of the few times in his life when he had talked openly about his illness, I expressed surprise, asking why he did not share his plight with medical colleagues, especially psychiatrists. He told me it just wasn't done and that "you'd stop getting referrals." How unfortunate that a profession presumably dedicated to care cannot extend compassion to one of its own! Other doctors shared similar stories:

> Society overall doesn't really accept it, let alone the medical profession. I mean, I can tell you that in my life story, that I was basically trashed because the hospital did not want to deal with somebody that had my diagnosis. And so they basically did what they needed to do. I basically was trashed. My career was ruined. (female physician, aged 46)

> I go to a physician support group, and they were talking about how there was a group of surgeons and one of the surgeons came down with cancer and had to start slacking off on the amount of work that this person did. And all the partners were grumbling and being upset about the fact that they had to take up the slack. And they may have expressed concern, but it didn't come out in their behavior, you know. And mental illness . . . I mean, a physician with mental illness is considered impaired. I mean, it's tantamount to being an addict. So it's like okay for laymen to have mental illness, but it's not okay for a doctor to have it. (male physician, aged 44)

The dominant theme of this chapter—and really the motivating force of this book—is that everyone needs a forum for telling stories. In the next chapter I give special attention to children, who, by virtue of their age, rarely have a say in issues of medication. Given that increasing numbers of children are being treated with drug therapy for emotional and behavioral disorders, it only seems right that we hear directly from them what it is like to be young, suffering, and medicated.

Chapter 6

Teens Talk

I think a lot of kids . . . would say they share the opinion that they are definitely puppets on a string, that they really don't have any say. They don't really get to do anything outside of "Take your damn meds" and that is about it. . . . You don't have a choice. I am just going to say that either way the adult always wins. Yeah, the adult always has the last word.

—Matthew, high school
junior, aged 17

As any young person between the ages of thirteen and nineteen can attest, the teenage years are marked by confusion and inconsistent messages from society. Though physiologically ready for sexuality, young adults are told to be chaste. Though able-bodied, they are confined to part-time jobs. Treated as children one moment, they are called upon to fight wars the next. Many young people have found that, caught in an adult world that largely dictates the rules of their daily lives, "being a teenager isn't an identity, but a predicament most people live through."[1]

Teens must differentiate themselves from their parents and establish their own identities. They face the formidable task of negotiating a "balance of independence and dependence, autonomy and reliance on others, distance and closeness, change and stability."[2] Yet their efforts to discover their authentic selves are circumscribed by an educational system that dictates *where* young adults must be and *when, how* their after-school time is structured, and *what* life expectations and aspirations they ought to have for themselves.

The ways adolescents view illness and medication make sense only in the context of the social structures that define their lives. Each of the ten stories collected for this chapter involves students' experiences at school.[3] As their conversations will show, teenagers today struggle with a sense of powerlessness, alienation from adult authority, and competition for respect.

When people feel powerless, they construct social worlds where status, respect, and identity are governed by rules of their own making.[4] Teenagers are no different. During the teen years, the opinions of one's peers become crucial in shaping tastes, attitudes, and behaviors. Where a teen fits in the hierarchy of adolescent cliques significantly determines his or her self-esteem and emotional well-being. Respect is gained or lost through inclusion and exclusion. Among the worst fates for teenagers is to feel friendless or to be rejected by groups important to them. As I learned through my interviews, school can become a torturous place for teenagers who do not fit in.

Adolescence is especially difficult for emotionally troubled teens. Nearly always, manifestations of emotional distress such as excessive shyness, withdrawal, irritability, irrational anger, and, in the most extreme case, psychosis relegate sufferers to the youth culture's social equivalent of Siberia. Moreover, children identified as emotionally troubled find themselves under the gaze of adult authority just as they are trying to escape it. Teens struggling with emotional problems are often forced into a world of psychiatrists, therapists, and school counselors whose demands further mark them as different.

Parents and professionals dealing with emotionally disturbed children often describe their experiences as exhausting, frustrating, and challenging. So much of what teenagers do seems irrational and counterproductive from the perspective of adults. Distraught parents ask, "Why can't I get my child to see a psychiatrist?" "Why does she dye her hair purple and choose to hang out with her Goth friends?" "Why does she refuse to listen to anything I say?" "Why has taking medication become such a battle between us?" In this chapter I explore adolescent behavior from the other side: from the perspectives of the teens themselves in the contexts of their daily lives. The relative powerlessness of young people dramatically blunts their voices. It only seems fair that they be given a chance to talk about their experiences.

Stressing Out

I remember hearing the claim that the most dangerous place to be is in your own home. Once you factor in child abuse, violence between adult partners, and serious accidents such as burns and bathroom falls, it becomes clear that many people are safer on highways, working as police officers, or walking in high-crime areas than just sitting at home. After listening to teenagers' stories, I am inclined to make another contrarian claim: Schools that are expected to act *in loco parentis,* to educate children, to refine their sensibilities, and to provide a safe haven from a dangerous world are, in fact, extremely hazardous to the health of some young people. Emotional problems that children bring to school are often greatly exacerbated there. The combination of academic and social pressure can be distressing for even the most well-adjusted teen.

The students I talked to often described themselves as overwhelmed by the workload, the constant pressure of standardized exams, the arbitrariness of some teachers, and, of course, the anxiety associated with getting into college.[5] Complaining about the constant battery of exams, one young man told me:

> It's not making me a happy camper, really, that
> they're using us to make themselves look good. If we
> do badly on the test we get in trouble. But if we do really
> good on the test the teacher gets a pat on the
> back and we just sit there. What does that say? That
> would make anyone angry.

He also said:

> I first experienced all the stress in the seventh grade,
> when I had to deal with massive amounts of projects.

I thought I was depressed because I was just getting whacked [with work]. (Andrew, eighth grade, aged 14)

One young woman described how academic expectations had intensified her emotional problems:

I would be sitting in class and feel really anxious, sometimes to the point of tears, and not really knowing why. And not sad tears but just scared, like, "Oh my God, what is going on?" I just felt overwhelmed all the time and really anxious. I remember it in sophomore year . . . just because . . . school started becoming difficult. I couldn't really concentrate in class, which would contribute to the anxiety, or sometimes the anxiety would be the reason why I couldn't concentrate. My homework started to become extremely difficult to me. . . . I would have different assignments in English class and just agonize over it, and the writing and not knowing where to start, how to start, not thinking I could do it. (Carol, college sophomore, aged 19)

Others responded to the demands of school by acting out. A sixteen-year-old girl whose life centered on an older crowd, illicit drugs, and weekend raves explained, "I just started not caring about it [school]. It was something I had to do. At fourteen I just started hating it."[6] A bright and articulate high school junior told me, "I stayed behind at least two years. I had four years in the seventh grade. . . . I wasn't doing my work. I just didn't care." A fif-

teen-year-old boy diagnosed with attention deficit hyperactivity disorder (ADHD), a diagnosis he denied, felt bad
about his poor grades but resented the many "speeches"
he had to endure:

> You have a meeting. They talk about . . . everything
> that is wrong with you. . . . They give you lectures
> about how you can do better and stuff like that. I had
> so many of those lectures and speeches it is not even
> funny. . . . They tell you the same speeches over and
> over and over [and] you get sick of hearing it after a
> while. They try to embed it in your head. It gets on
> your nerves hearing the same speech over and over
> and over.

More distressing for most teens than academic expectations is the pressure to fit in, to be accepted and valued by
one's peers. When the sociologist Murray Milner asked
teenagers, "Which would you rather do, flunk a test or eat
alone in the cafeteria?" most said they would rather flunk
a test.[7] While students have relatively little power in a
world controlled by adults, Milner notes, "in one realm
their power is supreme; they control their evaluations of
one another. That is, the kind of power they do have is
status power."[8] An eleventh-grade girl put it simply: "I
think just one main component to teenage depression . . .
is your peers. . . . In high school it's all about the friends
you have."

The need to fit in often leads to pettiness and vindic-
tiveness. Merciless teasing and put-downs are common-

place as teens at all levels of the status system struggle to differentiate themselves from those lower in the hierarchy.[9] Adults often view adolescents as overly sensitive, unnecessarily self-conscious, and hypervigilant. Yet such characteristics are necessary to operate within a tenuous and volatile status system. Even small missteps can have devastating consequences for teens' emotional health. One student suffering from an anxiety disorder called trichotillomania (compulsive hair pulling) traced the start of the problem to an event in middle school:

> I've been always playing with my hair since I was little, and in middle school, it was hell for anyone. . . . I remember one event. At my school there was a big brown or white day, where there's a big basketball tournament between the brown and white teams. Those were our school colors and I remember I was cheering for white. I was in the wrong section and I didn't realize that. And I got sort of laughed off. . . . And I go running out, go to the library, and pull out all of my eyelashes. So that was the big start. (Mia, college freshman, aged 19)

Although the teens I interviewed acknowledged that there were many nice people at school, they explained that they were easily overshadowed by those who were "out for blood." One eighth-grader told me: "Don't get me wrong, there are a lot of good people in the school. I've spent my whole life at [this school]. I know pretty much everybody in the school. I know when a person is going to make fun of who you are and what's wrong. If a person has a weakness, some of them just know how to exploit it." He explained: "My emotions just kind of went wild [after my parents' divorce]. For that I was teased by my peers. . . . I'm so easy to piss off, as they say. . . . It's not easy when people are saying that you are this wild maniac that can't control his emotions." In a world where looking cool and unfazed is highly valued, students with significant emotional problems fare badly:

> I was sad a lot. I would start crying a lot. . . . I was afraid that [kids] would cast me out. I didn't know if they would understand or not. I didn't really want to scare anybody, either. I didn't want them to push me away . . . because I was trying to fit in so really bad. I felt like I was alone in the world and that nobody knew exactly what was happening. I didn't want to deal with anything. I didn't want to deal with the laughing at school. . . . In class people are like, what are you staring at? And they joke about it. What are you, schizophrenic? At lunchtime people would come up to me [and say], "What's your problem? Are you insane?" One time this girl, she was younger than me, I was in the eighth grade and she was in the sixth, she came up to me [and asked], "Are you a witch? Do you do witchcraft?" I was like, "No." And then they would come up to me with the rosary beads and they would be like this [makes a cross with her fingers]. It sym-

bolizes evil, Satan. They would say, "Oh, you're evil. Get back, you witch." They made references to voo-doo a lot. (Erica, sophomore, aged 16)[10]

Not surprisingly, young people will often go to great lengths to keep secret their use of psychiatric medications. Though there is now less stigma attached to psychotropic drug use in general, in the world of adolescents, being different can mean being labeled defective. It is true that relatively open talk about medications is possible in some schools, like the one described by a college freshman: "I went to one of those high schools in Washington, D.C., where a lot of elite parents send their kids. There's a lot of depression among kids that requires them to see the nurse to take pills." Even in this case, though, there were distinctions among pills. He continued: "I think kids do share with each other, but for some reason Ritalin and that stuff [for ADHD] is more shared than Zoloft. It's okay to be ADD, but people don't want to talk about being depressed. . . . I see the kids taking antidepressants at school and there's something really wrong with them. . . . I didn't want to be a part of that group." Another student, after acknowledging that his friends "semi-know about me," told me that "not many people find it [taking psychiatric drugs] a really attractive quality." Others added:

It would change a lot of things [if people knew I took medications]. People would think of me differently.

People would think that I was this out-of-control guy that can't live without this medication. People would think that I'm trying to keep it subtle here but I can't, that I freak. And that's something that I just don't want to deal with. I've dealt with enough crap in my lifetime to deal with that. (Andrew, eighth grade, aged 14)

It gives the other people the sense that there is something really wrong with you. It makes people think that you're insane. . . . It is just the comments that they make because I have a tendency to retaliate and argue back. I would never punch anybody. I am not violent but I would retaliate. (Erica, sophomore, aged 16)

They [kids on medications] get made fun of. People call them retarded and stuff. They are a step down [socially]. They feel like, "I am in trouble." Yeah, I am pretty sure a lot of kids don't want people to know they are on medication, especially nerdy kind of kids. If they are kind of nerds, that would add way more problems to their lives. [It would] make things more complicated. (Robert, freshman, aged 15)

Given that teenagers are so sensitive about their medication use, you would think that schools might respect their need for privacy. The young people I interviewed explained that medications are often administered by the school nurse. Rather than discreetly being given their pills, students are often summoned to the nurse's office over a loudspeaker. Having your name called and then having to conspicuously leave the classroom amounts to a "public degradation ceremony," since, according to my interviewees, everyone knows the purpose of the trip.[11] As a fifteen-year-old boy named Robert explained:

> I don't think it is cool to take medication. . . . It's just one of those things that get in your way. I used to have to take it during lunchtime. The nurse calls you down [and] that would be embarrassing. If you have to go to the nurse's office and take your medication, they call you over the intercom. They'd be like, "Somebody, somebody please come to the nurse's office," and everybody knows what it is for—medication.

One of the most powerful measures of student alienation and stress is the need to escape school altogether. One student who was essentially "doing her time" described how she used her illness to make periodic "jail breaks":

> They have cops at the exits. If they know you are skipping school, they won't let you out. So we just put two friends in the trunk and we would pull out. I start crying. I am like, "I have to go home. I have emotional problems." [The police] would let us go and I would stop crying and start laughing. It was a funny experience. (Ashley, freshman, aged 16)

More troubling still, several of the teenagers were so distraught by their illnesses and the way they were treated at school that they had to drop out for a while and sometimes change schools. Two students even described hospitalization as a respite from school. One explained: "I wanted a break from school. I was like, 'Please put me in the hospital.'" For others, medication side effects made school unbearable:

> I was taken off Zyprexa . . . but I was still on Depakote. People were noticing my weight gain, and I wasn't happy about that. They were like, "Oh, you look different. It looks like your face is a little thicker." Yeah, I was like, "Thanks." I was getting really mad because my favorite pants weren't fitting. I was getting frustrated and I would cry. I would throw all my clothes around. I would say, "I am fat. I have nothing to wear." It just got worse over the summer, too. I started ninth grade. I was actually only there for a week and a half because I wanted to leave that school because of my weight. Because people were telling me, "Oh, wow, you look really different" in a kind of, "I feel bad for you but you look really disgusting" sort of way. (Erica, sophomore, aged 16)

Erica went to a different school but remained there only one day:

> I came home crying and refused to go back there because people started with me on the first day. It was

my weight. I had really baggy pants that I liked to wear. They came from this rock store called Hot Topic. You can tell a person stepped on my pants on purpose. They would be like, "Oops." They made fun of my necklace, which was the pentagram because [I was] into Wicca then. . . . They also made fun of my hair, which was kind of short. Kids can be . . . very crude and cruel. It is just really horrible.

As shown in earlier chapters, adults often resist taking psychotropic drugs because they are unwilling to place themselves in a devalued category. While respect is surely a building block of all communal life, the social equivalent of carbon in the natural world, it is particularly important in the lives of teenagers. Adults have more options for dealing with powerlessness and diminished respect in different areas of their lives. For example, respect lost at work might be regained within the context of the family, or vice versa.[12] For adolescents, by contrast, life revolves around a single institution—the school. Thus the respect and acceptance of their peers become their most important possession. We should expect that under this distinctive social arrangement teenagers will resist anything that robs them of vital cultural currency. When young people fight against psychiatric diagnoses and prescribed drugs, they are not simply being obstinate and uncomprehending. They are fighting for their social lives.

Managing Pill Pressure

What does it mean to be troubled? At what point does someone decide that a personal difficulty is sufficiently bothersome that something ought to be done about it? Coming to believe that you are a troubled person involves a predictable social process. At first people may feel only a diffuse unease that they define as temporary. As the discomfort persists, they may initiate conversations with family and friends in an effort to name the "problem" and to consider remedies. When informal solutions fail to resolve the difficulty, they may seek the advice of professional experts trained to offer diagnoses and suggestions for treatment.[13] The process, however, becomes volatile and messy when people disagree with those who claim that their difficulties are abnormal. Although some of the teenagers I spoke to were so ill that they clearly needed medical help, most felt that the difficulties they were experiencing were normal for their age group.

In nearly every case the push to pills came from parents and was met with resistance. At least initially, the basis for resistance was similar to that described by the adults in my study. One student said: "I was really against it. I felt like it would change me. I didn't really want to take medication." Another explained his fear that "if I take the pill I'm going to turn into a stone." In an apparent effort to calm his anxiety, this boy's parents told him only that he would be taking "antistress" pills. Yet another teen told me: "I don't like taking medications. They don't make you who you are. They change your personality." Despite sometimes prolonged resistance, these students eventually surrendered to their parents' wishes. The process often began with a soft sell: "They kept saying that nothing is going to change. 'You're going to be the same old goofy guy, but you're going to feel less stressed.'" Continued resistance, however, prompted more insistent prodding and lecturing from parents until the children finally relented:

> I was actually very angry when I found out they
> wanted me on medication. I was crying. Everybody,
> my parents, my psychiatrist, my clinicians at school,
> my counselor, wanted me on medication. I just kept
> saying no. I said, "I don't want them. I don't want my
> thinking process to go away. I need my thinking.
> That is how I survive." So I just kept saying, "No, I
> don't want them, I really don't want them." They
> were pressuring/lecturing. It was weird. They just told
> me . . . how I would feel better. Then I got sick of
> hearing it, so I gave in. (Erica, sophomore, aged 16)

Even after the teens capitulated, they often continued to exercise a measure of autonomy through partial compliance:

> Mom wants me to take it. I had to take it for Mom,
> but I didn't want to take it for me. So there was a lot
> of like, parent-child conflict in it. I lied a lot about
> taking it. My mom used to fill up one of those pill
> boxes and I was supposed to take it. What ended up

happening a lot is that I would take it a couple of days. And then the weekend would come and I wouldn't take it over the weekend. (Katy, college junior, aged 20)

I thought it was stupid, honestly. When somebody puts you on medication, everybody had to think there is something wrong with me. . . . When they first give you medication you don't want to take it. [My mother] would leave the pills by the computer in the morning so I would have to take it. I would just leave it there and just walk out and go to school. Then my mom would always yell at me after school. She would be like, "Why didn't you take your medication? You are supposed to take your medication every morning." I was like, "I ain't taking it. I don't need to take it. I don't want to take it." And then it would go back and forth for a while. Then I would just go into my room and close the door, put some music on. (Robert, freshman, aged 15)

Two of the students I interviewed attended an alternative high school for emotionally troubled teenagers. In both cases, their path to alternative education followed disastrous experiences in public middle or high schools. Unlike mainstream public high schools, theirs served only forty students and offered a wide range of therapeutic services. Though they still had to contend with the cruelty of neighborhood teenagers who labeled them "speds" (special education students), school for them was now a community, "a family [where] . . . we help each other out." Moreover, these two students were more accepting of their diagnoses and more willing to follow their prescribed drug regimens than the other teens I spoke with. Claire, a junior, described how she came to accept her illness and ultimately her self:

> For the longest time, I didn't tell anybody because I was afraid they wouldn't want to be my friend. . . . But then I said to myself, "It's me. If people find out that I have bipolar disorder, fine. It's me." I sort of realized that I didn't need to keep anything a secret. It's me, it's who I am. And it's not, "Mom, when friends come over you can't let them know that I take medicine." If they see a pill bottle, let them see a pill bottle, you don't have to hide everything. If they don't want to be my friend because I have something, that's fine. If they ask their parents what it is, and their parents have a problem with it, that's fine. I don't really care anymore. It's who I am. It's fine.

The question of compliance with medication regimens is a complicated one for sure: teens told me that they feared being labeled mentally ill, experiencing unpleasant side effects, and losing important parts of their personalities. Nonetheless, several young people said that the most difficult aspect of being on medication was remembering to take the pills:

I don't like remembering to take the pill in the morning. . . . Who is going to remember to take the pill every morning? (Robert, freshman, aged 15)

The worst thing is remembering because I can't. . . . I'll always forget. She'll [mother] ask [all the time], "Have you taken your pills? Have you taken your pills?" (Carolyn, junior, aged 17)

I used to always forget taking my drugs, and then my mom used to run after me with my pills. When I was on the bus it was sort of embarrassing. (Allen, college sophomore, aged 20)

Should we simply attribute such behavior to the general forgetfulness of teenagers? Perhaps. But then, as the following quote suggests, chronic forgetfulness may actually mark a passive-aggressive attitude toward psychiatric drugs:

I don't see [forgetting] as that serious. I mean . . . like, birth control pills . . . I'd be more sure to take it. . . . It's sort of a motivation that if I don't take [the antidepressants] for a couple of days I'll start getting really bad headaches. But if I'm laying in my bed and I think, "Oh, I haven't taken my pills" . . . it's sort of like a toss-up as to whether I'll get up and go take them or just go to sleep. (Carolyn, junior, aged 17)

Perhaps more than at any other time, the teen years raise a number of profound questions. What distinguishes the normal pain of living from the pathological pain of disease? At what point along a continuum of difficulty do we decide that a medical problem exists? To what degree are affective disorders normal responses to pathological social systems? Most of the teenagers I interviewed insisted that there was nothing wrong with them. While we might dismiss their claims to normalcy as yet another instance of teenage immaturity or denial, there are good reasons to listen to them. The line between adolescent angst and mental illness can be blurry.

Pain is a relative notion; we have no real way to measure it. Indeed, one of life's dilemmas is that we are ultimately alone with our pain. However, whether we determine that our pain is a problem to be solved hinges on our willingness to see it as inappropriate, as unexpected, as well beyond the boundaries of the difficulties experienced by others. It is an unhappy commentary on the lives of teenagers that they routinely view their lives as difficult and painful. One student spoke for many when she explained: "It sucks to be a teenager. I don't have a boyfriend. I hate my life. Depression is like just down there. . . . Everyone has it." As many teens see it, being labeled mentally ill and obligated to take pills only exacerbates a normal set of problems. For that reason, several teenagers had a powerful motive to reject their diagnoses:

> Aren't kids supposed to be energetic? Being hyped up and running around all the time? It was kind of

funny. . . . I just thought, "Hey, it's normal for me." I
thought it was normal, so why should I be on medications to calm down? . . . I thought being energetic
was cool. . . . When they tell you [that] you can't be
energetic and they try to put you on medication, it's
like, "Wow, what is this? What are you trying to do to
me?" (Robert, freshman, aged 15)

I never thought something wasn't right. My mom
thought something wasn't right. I didn't start taking
medication until tenth grade, and she noticed something wrong in the eighth grade. . . . They figured I
had dysthymia because of what my mom said . . . but
I never believed what she said was true. . . . I can see
[why my mother believed the diagnosis]. Like when
everything was going on with school I would come
home and sometimes cry or I would just leave
school. . . . I think my behavior can go up and down
once in a while, but I wouldn't admit that something
is wrong with me or that I need medication. (Alyssa,
junior, aged 16)

I think sometimes society wants you to think and act
a certain way. When you don't, they give you drugs
and that sort of makes you act that way. . . . I really
didn't think I needed it. . . . You've got to have your
ups and downs in life. That's what I thought. . . . I
didn't think I needed it. I didn't like being considered
depressed. . . . My mom is telling me, "Look, it's just
to help. You may not be depressed but it will help if

> depression creeps into you." . . . I don't know why
> people don't just lay off me and let me be a normal
> kid. (Allen, college sophomore, aged 20)

Denial seems a plausible response in the cases just described. More puzzling was teenagers' tendency to "normalize" very dramatic behaviors. One young man who had spent years in state care and had been hospitalized several times acknowledged that he "flips out" every now and then. At the same time he felt angry that he had "been smacked with a diagnosis." He explained: "I don't accept any diagnosis, really. I don't believe in diagnoses. If they want to diagnose me, fine, whatever. Have fun."

Some of the teens talked about cutting, or self-mutilation, as a way to ease their emotional pain. Girls especially spoke of the behavior as though it were routine and ordinary: "I was into the blood. I liked to see the blood. That was my relief. I loved the blood. It's like watching paint drip out of yourself, and it was my only relief." Another said: "To me, cutting was something completely different. To everyone else it was like, 'Well, if she's cutting, who knows what could happen next.'" Several girls noted that though they often saw the tell-tale signs of cutting on other students, the behavior was rarely discussed openly; when it was, most teens dismissed it as harmless. One high school junior gave this example: "I'd carve names and I'd say, 'Look, I carved my name into my leg.' And they'd say, 'Cool.' And I'd say, 'Yuh, it took me five minutes.' I'd make a joke about it, but inside it kind of hurt. . . . They'd just say, 'Oh, you made a tattoo.'"

Could it be that pain has become so much a part of adolescence that young people have difficulty distinguishing between normal and pathological behavior? In school
settings where violence is routine, drugs prevalent, pressures to conform unyielding, and humiliation the norm,
perhaps depression and anxiety are not easily separated
from "normal" teenage unhappiness. This emotional
blind spot, combined with the fear of being labeled mentally ill, can only deepen adolescent malaise. Teenagers,
consequently, deny the need for treatment until their
emotional problems become unendurable. Coerced into
taking pills they do not believe they need and would pre-
fer to avoid, they often respond with anger:

> Poetry is my outlet. All of my emotions go onto pa-
> per. . . . I feel that this has been taken away from me
> by medication. I would like to have control over my-
> self. I don't want the medications to have control
> over me. . . . I feel like I have been just lied to and just
> been used. I feel like an experiment actually with all
> the different medications they have used. I feel I have
> been used as a test subject. (Erica, sophomore,
> aged 16)

> I had an experience with Zoloft [in the hospital]. I am
> like, "Don't put me on Zoloft. . . . What are you guys
> giving me Zoloft for?" I went up to the desk and I am
> like, "Why did you give me Zoloft? Take that away." I
> knew they gave me Zoloft right after I took it. . . .
> When you're in a mental institution, bam! It's no dis-

cussion. "You can call my doctor. I guarantee he will tell you the same exact thing. I am horrible with Zoloft. I am a friggin' nut job. Don't give me Zoloft." They ended up calling the doctor after I flipped out and had the seizure. He was like, "Yep, he doesn't do well on Zoloft. He flips out." They are like, "Oh, really." (Matthew, junior, aged 17)

Given the stigma attached to psychiatric drugs among adolescents and the fact that they often fail to work, it makes sense that some teens would choose to self-medicate with alcohol and street drugs. In their world, alcohol and marihuana, especially, have clear advantages over prescribed medications. These drugs, in stark contrast to antidepressants, are typically used during collective events that foster solidarity and friendship among teens. The pressure to participate in their use is not seen as an imposition of power and control. Caught between adult demands that they take their medicine and the desire to party with their friends on weekends, the teens I talked to sometimes experimented with their prescribed drugs and alcohol:

I had a lot of creativity, and it felt great to be manic that first twelve to eighteen hours where I would get this rush. If I were to take the medications Monday through Thursday night, I stopped taking them on Friday. By Friday night I could start on my upward trend. It was my upward trend on Friday and Saturday and then my Sunday crash. . . . And especially if I would drink on the weekends, that would just send me into the real low pits. But I just figured that Sunday night was the night before you have to go back to school on Monday. And everyone has bad Sunday nights, right? (Katy, college junior, aged 20)

One high school freshman whose use of ecstasy eventually resulted in severe anxiety nevertheless unfavorably compared psychiatric drugs with recreational drugs:

I don't regret doing [ecstasy]. I did too much. Let's put it that way. It really gives you a different perspective on life. Well, they each have side effects, let's put it that way. [A lot of] side effects. But the drugs psychiatrists give you, they don't make you think in such a positive way. They never made me think in a positive way. [But] when . . . I was on E [ecstasy] you couldn't see a happier person. I would run up to people in the street and just talk to them and make them laugh. I gave a kid a green balloon one time. He was the happiest little kid you will ever find. It just brings out the better in everybody. You learn from that. You learn a lot from drugs, just the experimentation of it all. They are more valuable to me than the ones from psychiatrists. (Ashley, freshman, aged 16)

Ashley turned her back on school in order to hang out with friends whose lives also centered on drugs. In the delicate world of teenage standards this decision placed her in the category of "druggies." To protect herself and to maintain a modicum of respect, she defined herself as "more mature" than others and as "needing to be around people who have a different perspective on things." Teens who find themselves ostracized from the most popular groups at school often completely redefine their status hierarchies. They flaunt their uniqueness and scorn conventionality.

Finding Friends

We all have times when we feel our identity is threatened. For most of us, the damage is slight and has no lasting impact. We might, for example, suffer a moment of unexpected embarrassment that quickly fades from memory. In high school, by contrast, identity attacks are daily occurrences designed to regulate the status system. Put-downs, social slights, and hurtful gossip help keep students in their "rightful" place in the power structure. In such an unfriendly world most teens have simple goals: either to sustain their social position or to improve it. But for those who are tagged as different, including those with emotional problems, such goals are usually unattainable. They are often seen as permanently tainted.[14]

In response to being ostracized, virtually all the students I interviewed formed friendship groups that provided the comfort of like-minded people and an ideology that challenged the value structure that prevailed in their schools.[15] However much they may have tried to avoid diagnoses and medications, they fell into the problematic category of "emotionally troubled teens." In a context where belonging is everything, they reacted by forming countercultural friendship groups that celebrated their identities. The drift toward a new group of friends invariably began with rejection:

> When I was younger, like eight or ten, I had a lot of friends. But toward junior high, I had very few friends. . . . They treat kids horrible there. If you're a nerd or you dress a certain way that's not up to date, they'll pick on you so bad. If your hair is wrong they'll pick on you. . . . The school is so tough. We didn't have a lot of money back then, our family. I used to have to wear my mother's old clothes. The kids used to make fun of me because of that. . . . There's certain cliques. There's the popular clique, then there's the Puerto Rican clique or the Asians. And then there's the nerdy clique, and that's where I would fall. . . . People would just whisper about the way I dressed and the way I acted. They would just make fun of me. It was pretty bad. Sometimes I would come home and even cut myself. (Elaine, junior, aged 17)

> I never had any friends growing up. They always picked on me. I was never chubby. . . . but [I was] the ugly little girl with the big flippy hair. . . . In Catholic school it is really judgmental. If you don't look exactly like them you are not cool enough and what not. It was just really upsetting. (Ashley, freshman, aged 16)

I just started crying for no reason. So I went down to see my guidance counselor. I was just crying. After that I went down every day crying. Everyone started to know what was happening. They'd start talking about me and they would make fun of it. I was like, "Wow, this is so wrong." I just got really frustrated. . . . I would go home and cry. I would just be really upset by it, and some of these people used to be my friends. It just goes to show you who your real friends are. . . . I felt really betrayed, basically. (Erica, sophomore, aged 16)

Some teenagers were distressed when their circle of friends broke up, usually during the transition from middle school to high school:

Eighth grade, socialwise, was like great. I had a boyfriend and we had this group that was like four girls and four boys, and we jokingly referred to ourselves as "the collective" because we did everything together. We would get together and have movie nights. It was sort of the time when everyone started making out, so . . . just everyone would sit on the couch and make out/watch a movie. So it was really secure, like the eight of us. . . . Then it all started to break up over the summer. [When] freshman year started we were sort of together, but most of the couples had broken up. . . . And then freshman year sucked a lot. That was like the worst year. . . . I don't know . . . maybe it was partly the collective breaking up and not having the same close-knit group of friends. (Carolyn, junior, aged 17)

While most of the young people I interviewed were unwilling to embrace the idea that they were sick, they often recognized that they did not feel the same as their peers. Eager to fit in, they often went for years denying the feelings they had and pretending to have feelings they didn't. One girl explained that, as early as the fifth grade, "I wanted to be happy . . . [but] I felt like I was faking emotions. I could only reach a certain point and beyond that I was faking it. . . . I could be in a good mood, but as far as being 'Oh my God, this is fun, how great this is!' I felt like I was always pushing it." At a point, many of the teenagers realized that their friends had no idea what they were actually feeling, and pretending to be happy had simply become too emotionally taxing. Consequently, several withdrew from their circle of friends, mostly after they started to take medications. They now occupied two worlds that they believed were inaccessible to their friends—one emotional and the other medical:

> They [pills] made me different. I couldn't feel emotions. They just made me feel numb. . . . Thirteen and fourteen it was scary. No other people my age are dealing with that yet. They are just happy riding bicycles in circles down the street. . . . It is just really weird taking medication at that age. I couldn't talk to my friends about it because they have no idea what I am talking about. (Ashley, freshman, aged 16)

> It turns out that there were a lot of other different
> students who were going through different things.
> Some of them were diagnosed with depression and a
> lot of different things, [but at the time] it just felt like
> I was so alone. And even after I had been diagnosed
> and the psychologist would say there are a lot of peo-
> ple dealing with this, I just felt like, "No, no one else
> is going through what I'm going through." That's
> just how it feels. (Carol, college sophomore, aged 19)

Distressed, different, devalued, and often acutely lonely, adolescents are on the lookout for peers who might understand them and provide some solace. The first discovery is sometimes a single friend who speaks the same language. Ashley, a sophomore, said: "I had this one friend, her name is Vicki. . . . She is a lot like me. We don't try to sit around and be depressed. We try to be normal, I guess, and do normal things and have fun. It is really cool to have someone who is the same type of person. Some-times it gets a little too depressing [but] it kind of helps in a certain way." Other teens learned the hard way that many young people share their experience. Sixteen-year-old Erica described her first hospitalization: "It was ac-tually pretty exciting because I got to meet kids my age who had the same problems. I felt like I wasn't alone in the world. . . . It was really a joyous feeling . . . not excited in being there but in knowing I wasn't alone." The experi-ence of being with others who are also struggling emo-tionally usually leads young people to seek out even more kindred souls.

Depression and medication use are rarely the only bases for forming new friendships. Rather, the main criterion for membership is that people do not fit into conventional cliques. In characterizing their current friendship groups, students proudly described the members as "weird," "misfits," "outcasts." Listen to the way these groups were formed:

> Our old friends had dumped us and we didn't really have friends. We weren't really similar at all but we banded together. (Carolyn, junior, aged 17)

> I realized that I didn't need to fit in to be happy. That was just making it worse because I wasn't being myself. . . . I actually found some pretty good friends who were pretty much outcasts. (Erica, sophomore, aged 16)

> There is a little group of people called the "us" group. This is just a little clique that we have. Yeah, we're a bunch of people who are completely different. (Andrew, eighth grade, aged 14)

These groups provide a forum where otherwise taboo topics like depression can be openly discussed since "it's sort of accepted, like almost taken for granted that you're all depressed. . . . I mean, we joke about it. We'll be like, 'Oh yeah, what are you on?' And, 'Oh yeah, I forgot to take my medication today.'" More significant, these groups provide a philosophical perspective for turning the prevailing status hierarchy on its head.

Whenever I interview people about mental illness I ask them if anything good has come out of an otherwise negative experience. Nearly everyone responds that their suffering has made them more aware, more sensitive, and often more insightful than others. In much the same way, disenfranchised teens collectively produce a group ideology that expresses, in fact, a kind of elitism. Together, they use their negative attributes as the basis for declaring themselves superior to those who reject them. Unlike their peers who fit solidly into one or another favored clique and unthinkingly abide by the rigid social conventions of high school life, nearly all the teenagers with whom I spoke saw themselves and their friends as "deeper," as better understanding the value of diversity, and as more in touch with the profound complexities of life. The contrast is with other students who act like robots, comfortably insulated within their provincial social worlds and only dimly understanding the real stuff of life:

> There's a bunch of preppies that are just close-knit, and they do everything right and they're on the honor roll and in the newspaper and stuff. The ones that I'm friends with are like, on the border. [We're] not mainstream, I guess. [We're] different from most of the kids in high school. Like most of [my friends] have dyed hair. We don't really care much about fashion. [We wear] weird clothes. Nothing mainstream, just weird. . . . I think . . . they sort of gravitate toward

each other. They don't want to be normal like other people. They want to be different. And so they all get together and are different together. They're not willing to take things at face value and say, "Ok, this is what the world is like." We have really deep discussions. They write poetry and, I mean, they certainly aren't superficial. (Carolyn, junior, aged 17)

There's like three levels of uniqueness. There's not unique at all. There's like this kind of guy who's just different. Me, I'm the third level. I am just this completely different individual, and you know what? I am proud of it. I remember hearing this phrase from a friend of mine, who says, "You laugh at me because I'm different. I laugh at you because you're all the same." We are just not conformists. Like, we have this girl who is this brilliant, brilliant person. There's another person who is just really, really an oddball. And there is another girl who is another oddball. And there's just plenty of oddballing to go around. (Andrew, eighth grade, aged 14)

Everyone in seventh grade was going through the "how-deep-am-I phase." I went Goth. I shaved half my head, dyed it blue, lots of heavy eyeliner, black clothing. At that point I didn't fight the meds thing, because it was, "Oh, look how depressed I am." It was very cool to listen to heavy industrial rock. I liked the look. . . . It's very, sort of, I don't want to say glamorous, but the very pale skin . . . just seemed to fit me,

kind of. I'm not athletic at all. I have no gross motor
skills. I like writing, which fits. You write long ballads
in gothic poetry and I did all that. And these people
were depressed all the time, and at that point I could
. . . say, "I'm depressed. Hey, let's have a party." (Mia,
college freshman, aged 19)

I was somewhat surprised to find that "having problems" was not always a cause for status loss. Indeed, as
some teens explained, there was a certain cachet to having
emotional difficulties. A nineteen-year-old girl who was
diagnosed with depression in grade school remembered
telling her friends: "I don't think I really got it for a while.
Either I didn't tell them at all . . . or I said [whispering],
'Can you keep a secret? I'm diagnosed as depressed.' It did
separate me. It made me distinct. There is something
melodramatic about having issues." Another student told
me, "I was originally hospitalized for anorexia when I was
eleven or twelve, and I think being labeled as anorexic was
a positive label. Like, 'I'm anorexic and I have this huge
control over myself.'" Yet again, the boundary between
normalcy and pathology melts away under the glare of intense cultural pressures. As oppressive as unattainable
beauty standards might be, young women cannot easily
withstand them.[16] In certain domains, at least, illness is
understood as an appropriate and acceptable effort to
fit in.

The adolescents were creative in their attempts to solve,
or at least live with, their status problems. The formation
of alternative groups that reject majority standards is a

perfectly sensible way to deal with otherwise diminished identities. Like everyone else, teenagers believe that outsiders cannot understand what they are going through, and so they are resistant to external efforts to impose solutions. Aren't most of us distrustful, even resentful, of gratuitous advice offered by those who we believe have no real comprehension of our lives? As we have seen, teens typically view diagnoses and psychiatric drugs as adult solutions that do not accord well with their daily realities. In this light, perhaps what adults often call teenage recalcitrance might more properly be understood as a rejection of inappropriately applied adult power and illegitimate claims to expertise.

Dealing with Professional Authority

I once heard power defined as "the capacity to make someone do what you want them to do even if they don't want to do it." Authority, by contrast, resides in the belief that you should do what others want you to do because they have the right to tell you to do it.[17] Coercion is at the core of power while legitimacy is the source of authority. It follows that systems based on actual or perceived power are inherently less stable than those rooted in authority. While the teenagers I interviewed respected the authority of many adults, they often saw adult claims to legitimate authority over their lives as expressions of raw power. They regularly voiced disdain for professionals who, in their view, did not understand them, rarely helped them, treated them as incompetent, and further undermined their tenuous social positions among their peers. The ceaseless and arbitrary exercise of power bred anger and sometimes rebellion:

> I had a couple of teachers that I really liked. They were really cool. The others were just like [awful]. . . . One guy wouldn't even let me use the bathroom the whole class. I would just walk out. Screw you. I am using the bathroom. They thought I was going to do something terrible when I went to the bathroom. . . . Other guys would go in and smoke pot in the bathroom. I was like . . . all I have to do is use the toilet. They would walk me to the bathroom. They held the door for me. They treated me like I was incompetent. (Ashley, freshman, aged 16)

Holden Caulfield, the sixteen-year-old protagonist of J. D. Salinger's novel *The Catcher in the Rye,* speaks to teens who resent being labeled by authority figures.[18] Angry at the phoniness of adults, Caulfield pays the price for his uncompromising nonconformity. A chronic failure in school, he is considered disturbed and spends time in a psychiatric hospital. At one point Caulfield tries to explain himself to a school official: "'Look, sir. Don't worry about me,' I said. 'I mean it. I'll be all right. I'm just going through a phase right now. Everybody goes through phases and all, don't they?'"[19] A student I interviewed also spoke for most of his peers when he said: "I told them, 'Why do I need to see a therapist? . . . I'm not crazy or anything.' They try to be like, 'Don't worry, it's not because you're crazy. . . . It's just that you have to go.'"

Teenagers are justified in questioning the expertise of adult authorities; after all, the everyday world of adolescence changes significantly from generation to generation. The teens with whom I spoke rejected the legitimacy of therapists' right to treat them solely on the basis of professional expertise:

> I don't really want to talk to therapists. . . . I don't feel that they completely understand. They read books, but they don't go through it. (Ashley, freshman, aged 16)

> He didn't seem to understand. He was always really, really happy. He probably didn't understand anything I was saying. (Erica, sophomore, aged 16)

> I don't trust counselors. I don't like to sit down in a room and be questioned. I would never have started counseling unless my mom made me. (Alyssa, junior, aged 17)

Distrust eventually breeds resentment:

> I had to see someone to get the medication. So to me, whenever I had to go see him I would basically say to myself, "Okay, I have to go see him, but it's just because I need medicine, for no other reason." . . . I didn't like his style. I just felt like he was kind of arro-

gant. His claim to fame was that he worked with a lot of teenagers going through different things and so he really understood. But he didn't understand me. He didn't at all, and he thought he did. And that's one of my biggest pet peeves, when people think that they know me, and think that they know what's going on, and they just don't. (Carol, college sophomore, aged 19)

They don't know what they are talking about. Psychiatrists definitely don't know what they are talking about. All they do is sit there and doodle on their pads, or something. . . . The next time I come back, they are like, "So, how are we doing?" It is like, "Hello. . . . What were you writing down last time?" Yeah, I used to say that. "What were you writing down last time?" . . . Yeah, I think they doodle on their pad. I think they are writing little doodles. At one point I was seeing five or six psychologists or whatever. I don't know why. I don't know why they were making me see all these different people. I am like, "What is up with this?" (Matthew, junior, aged 17)

I hate it. I think it is a waste of time. It cuts into your life. . . . Yeah, it gets on your nerves. . . . You have to sit there for like an hour. . . . They just sit there and talk to you for an hour. Who likes that? . . . I mean, [being in] the office for a whole hour just talking to somebody. Yeah, it cuts into your life. I just told my caseworker I hate therapy. I don't want to go into it.

> She was like, "Well . . . you don't have a choice." Like
> my caseworker, she forced me . . . to go to therapy. I
> was forced to do that. (Robert, freshman, aged 15)

Children are in a particularly vulnerable position when dealing with mental health professionals. In earlier chapters we heard adults complain that too many doctors are paternalistic and withhold critical information from them. In such cases we are properly outraged on their behalf, but what about when the patients are children? Parents and mental health providers tell teenagers that a particular treatment or therapy is for their own good, and as a result they often feel tricked and lied to: "I feel like I have been just lied to and . . . been used. I feel like an experiment with all the different medications that have been used. I feel like I have been used as a test subject."

One compelling example of the connections among medications, feelings, and emotional development came from my interview with a college freshman. Diagnosed with depression at age eleven, Mia had been prodded into taking the antidepressant Zoloft by her mother, a therapist. When we talked, the young woman was still resentful toward her mother for having forced the issue. The resentment remained, in part, because neither her parents nor her doctors had ever explained the potential side effects of Zoloft, a prominent one being diminished libido. It was not until Mia was sixteen that a therapist revealed that her lack of sexual feelings was caused by the medication. This one conversation helped to explain years of anguish. She felt that as a result of being uninformed she had missed an important stage of adolescent development:

> So I went into therapy [at age sixteen] and found out
> a lot about the medication I was on for the first time.
> I heard the things I didn't know about Zoloft that no
> one ever bothered telling an eleven-year-old . . . which
> explained a whole hell of a lot. Because . . . I never
> went through a phase, you know, when you're about
> twelve or thirteen and you start to notice boys. I had
> never gone through that. . . . I didn't have that. And I
> thought for years, "Oh my God, am I gay, am I asex-
> ual?" I had no idea. And no one was telling me maybe
> your pills have something to do with it. . . . I had no
> sex drive, no libido, and I'd never gone through the
> phase where everyone starts to notice boys. So I guess
> about fifteen or sixteen that just totally made a whole
> hell of a lot of sense. Because for a while I thought I
> was gay because of the absence of any attraction to-
> ward boys. Or, rather, it would be sort of a quick
> burst. It's like, "Oh, he's cute, yeah." That was it. So I
> was like, "What the hell is going on?" And I'd say,
> "Okay, I'm just asexual. Christ, that sucks." And [my
> doctor] . . . [finally] said, "No, this is one of the big
> symptoms, one of the big problems people have with
> SSRIs. Maybe you should go off of them." It's the
> first time a doctor had . . . given me an alternative.

The students I interviewed longed to turn eighteen, the
age of legal adulthood. At eighteen they could enter the

labor force, move away from home, and, if they wished, stop treatments they thought had been inappropriately imposed on them. The case was most explicitly made by Andrew, a seventeen-year-old who strongly identified with his Irish heritage: "I'm pretty much thinking of getting off [medications] when I turn eighteen. I'm going to be an adult." Stopping pills, however, was only one part of his plan. Andrew imagined moving to Ireland, changing his name, and leaving behind all the painful experiences that had colored his life thus far:

> One of the things I am trying to do when I leave [for Ireland], I am trying to leave behind my whole iden-tity. . . . I am trying to go so nobody knows me. It is starting off a new life, that's it. . . . I am going to change my first name.

> *You are literally going to become reborn?*

> Yep, like [I want to forget] the hospitalization . . . ev-erything. If I do have kids I don't want them to have to deal with all that. . . . I just want to get rid of every-thing. I don't really like the stuff that happened to me. Bad history. I had a really screwed-up infancy, let's just say it that way. . . . If I have kids I don't want them to grow up that way.

Andrew, like some of the other teens, was hoping that adulthood would expand his opportunities to fashion a new identity. His story and others' have shown that the way adolescents respond to emotional troubles and medication use is linked to their relative powerlessness and to the demands of a school world that has little tolerance for those who do not meet rigid standards. Their thoughts and feelings, just as with adults, cannot be separated from the social world they inhabit and the demands it makes of them.

Thus far I have focused on the connections between psychiatric medications and *personal* identity. Next I will consider how our *collective* cultural identity is being shaped by the movement toward biological thinking in psychiatry. The last chapter will address the radical implications of psychiatry's increasing power over our minds and emotions and, thereby, over our ideas about what it means to be happy and well.

Chapter 7

High on Drugs

*On Prozac, Sisyphus might well push the boulder back up the
mountain with more enthusiasm and more creativity. I do
not want to deny the benefits of psychoactive medication. I
just want to point out that Sisyphus is not a patient with a
mental health problem. To see him as a patient with a mental
health problem is to ignore certain larger aspects of his predicament connected to boulders, mountains, and eternity.*

—Carl Elliott, *Better Than*
Well, p. 160

Biological psychiatry, with its claim to an expanding
number of psychiatric brain diseases requiring medical
treatment, has fundamentally redefined the meanings we
attach to our own feelings. In this last chapter I will consider some of the disturbing cultural implications of psychiatry's new pill paradigm.[1]

The best evidence we have at the moment is that
schizophrenia, major depression, and manic depression
have significant biological components.[2] Although scientists have not been able to determine the exact role of

brain chemistry in such disorders, we do know that psychotropic medications can help diminish human suffering. Surely, scientists and pharmaceutical companies should continue to investigate how brain lesions, faulty neurotransmitter processes, and flawed genes might shape thoughts and feelings that severely impair human functioning. At the same time, by insisting that affective disorders are primarily caused by malfunctioning brains, biological psychiatry ignores clear evidence about the psychological and social factors at the core of human emotions.[3] The more people embrace the view, unrelentingly pushed by pharmaceutical companies and some doctors, that their feelings are symptoms of diseases to be treated with pills, the greater the risk to personal autonomy and responsibility.

Our ideas about what constitutes diseases, the kinds of treatments we then seek for our emotional problems, and the care that is extended to us are all contingent on how we view pain and pathology. Consider, as well, that ideas about illness and treatment are shaped by powerful organizations seeking to maximize profits. Patients can receive care only for conditions recognized by insurance companies, and HMOs offer only those treatments that *appear* most cost-effective. The view that negative feelings require biochemical intervention affects simultaneously the lives of individuals and the life of a society. The anthropologist T. M. Luhrmann describes well the double-edged implications of psychiatry's shift from a psychodynamic to a biomedical model:

> The disease model of mental illness has been a tre-
> mendous asset in the fight against stigma and the
> fight for parity in health care coverage. And it is clear
> that the disease model captures a good measure of
> the truth. Mental illness often has an organic quality.
> People can't just pull themselves back together when
> they are hearing voices or contemplating suicide. . . .
> Yet to stop at that model, to say that mental illness is
> nothing but disease, is like saying that an opera is
> nothing but musical notes. It impoverishes us. It im-
> poverishes our sense of human possibility.[4]

Luhrmann has also observed that "a great ambiguity in psychiatry" is "Who owns a person's mental state? Who has the right to know it?"[5] Such questions are critical since human freedom may ultimately reside in our ability to think and feel things that are contrary to social convention. Even in the most oppressive circumstances people can retain a measure of integrity—indeed, sanity—by holding onto their thoughts, feelings, and sensibilities. We rely on the sacred preserve of our innermost thoughts to sustain our humanity. However, with the increasing acceptance of the biomedical model, we begin to believe that more and more of our feelings are illegitimate and abnormal, and require biological intervention to correct. There is a great loss in that.

As I write these words, well past America's "victory" in Iraq, our government and the soldiers on the ground are still trying to win the hearts and minds of the Iraqi people. This most recent military adventure illustrates yet again what wars and subsequent occupations always reveal: Subduing minds and feelings is always more complicated than subduing bodies. Analogously, the stories presented in this book show that while most patients ultimately surrender to drug therapy—believing, in the end, that they have little choice otherwise—they nearly always act as resistance fighters along the way. Resistance takes the form of failure to comply with doctors' orders, self-experimentation with drugs, and repeated efforts to stop taking the pills altogether. At its root is the sense that prescribed drugs can erode personal authenticity and deprive people of feelings that reflect their true selves. Yet the fact that so many patients eventually accept biological explanations of their problems indicates the speed with which biological psychology is gaining currency.

The Triumph of Biological Psychiatry

Years ago problematic behavior was explained simply as evidence of sinfulness or evil. This vocabulary of sinfulness has largely been superseded by a "sickness" vocabulary. These days when people behave strangely or do things that impinge on our moral sensibilities, we immediately question their mental health: "Why aren't these people acting normal?" "What's wrong with them?" Consequently, an ever-increasing variety of behaviors now fall under the rubric of the "medical model."

Although presumably based on objective scientific criteria thoroughly independent of moral judgments or political ideologies, the medical model conflates the idea of health with cultural conceptions of normalcy. In the name of science, the medical model unjustifiably gives physicians the right to "treat" behaviors that contravene social expectations or upset widely held moral injunctions. Examples of nonconforming behaviors[6] that have been medicalized include hyperactivity in children, child abuse, and alleged shopping, sexual, and computer addictions.[7] Despite claims to the contrary, science and morality are inseparably linked when medicine is accorded the right to define the causes and then the legitimate treatments for disturbing behaviors.

Psychiatric treatment of new illnesses has accelerated since the 1980s. Whereas psychiatry traditionally had been dominated by a psychodynamic perspective on illness, the field has turned its back on that tradition in favor of predominantly biological definitions of mental illness. Critics of this shift focus their attention on the social factors that have led psychiatrists to the prescription pad. One can only express wonderment at the "discovery" of so many new brain diseases since 1980. The bible of psychiatric diagnoses, the *Diagnostic and Statistical Manual of Mental Disorders,* or DSM, has now been revised three times since 1953, most recently in 1994.[8] The first two editions classified illnesses in accordance with the psychodynamic model prevalent at the time. Conditions warranting psychiatric treatment were understood as *disorders* of the *mind.* Then, in the 1980s, the language of psychotherapeutic disorder abruptly disappeared and was replaced by *diseases* of the *brain*. In 1953, the DSM named 60 psychiatric disorders. In 1969, the number of diagnostic categories had doubled to 120. In 1987 more than 200 diagnostic categories were listed. The current DSM describes over 350 diagnoses.[9]

Surely a 480 percent increase in the number of psychiatric abnormalities over fifty years cannot result solely from dispassionate scientific discovery. The transition from disorder to disease and the proliferation of such diseases are more a function of cultural, economic, and political processes than scientific advances. In fact, the sharpest critics of psychiatry's current stance maintain that, except for a few major psychotic illnesses, there is no evidence that the multiplication of conditions listed as brain diseases in the DSM warrant that designation.[10]

We often hear diagnoses from the DSM likened to organic conditions such as diabetes. The analogy breaks down, however, when we consider that no doctor would prescribe insulin replacement without first clearly demonstrating that a person's body was not properly producing the hormone. Doctors have a definitive test to affirm the organic pathology that warrants the diabetes diagnosis and, thus, subsequent treatment. By contrast, no doctor has ever done a diagnostic test that demonstrates the brain dysfunction for which I am prescribed my drugs. Like others treated with antidepressant medications, I am *presumed* to have a brain disease on the basis of the symptoms I report. The tenuous connections among symptoms, diagnoses, demonstrable physical pathologies, treatments, and outcomes undermine the validity of the disease model in psychiatry. As the psychiatrist Thomas Szasz writes:

> Asserting that a particular person's problem is a disease because the patient or others *believe* it is a disease, or because it looks like a disease, or because doctors *diagnose* it as a disease, and treat it with drugs as if it *were* a disease, or because it *entitles the subject to be qualified as disabled,* or because it *presents an economic burden to the subject's family or society*—all that is irrelevant to the scientific concept of disease.[11]

If psychiatry's radical and unwavering turn toward biology cannot be justified in terms of dispassionate medical research, how are we to understand the transformations I have been describing? In my view the turn to biology has occurred in part because it *is* unclear whether psychiatrists are, in fact, treating diseases. That is to say, psychiatry has always fought for legitimacy as a medical specialty. Consequently, psychiatrists have something to gain in terms of professional prestige if they can convince themselves and others that troubled people need their chemical interventions to heal broken brains just as someone with a broken leg needs an orthopedic surgeon. The impulse toward greater legitimacy also bears a synergistic relationship to the interests of pharmaceutical companies that make billions of dollars selling psychotropic medications. It is a perfect system. Pharmaceutical companies need diseases for their drugs. The American Psychiatric Association creates and codifies these diseases in the DSM. Finally, the more diseases patients bring to psychiatrists for treatment, the more their status is enhanced.

The stakes in getting a drug approved by the Food and Drug Administration (FDA) are high. In the case of psychiatric medications alone the numbers are staggering. In 2001, Americans spent more than 12 billion dollars on antidepressant medications, the equivalent of $43.85 for every man, woman, and child in the country.[12] In 1999 doctors in the United States wrote 24,742,000 prescriptions for Prozac alone, and thirty-eight million people worldwide have used the drug between 1988 and 2000.[13] Moreover, between 1987 and 1996 there was a two- to threefold increase in the number of American adolescents being treated with psychiatric medications.[14] Given the profits involved, it is easy to see that drug companies might go to great lengths to gain FDA approval for their pills and then to market them.

Indeed, numerous exposés demonstrate the way drug companies slant research findings and limit damaging information about drugs to both doctors and patients.[15] Researchers often subtly manipulate the data by choosing design strategies to ensure the greatest likelihood of showing a drug's effectiveness. Consequently, pharmaceutical companies deliberately adopt research approaches that cast the competition in a negative light. Technically these strategies are not illegal, but they are unquestionably unethical and ensure that patients never get the full story as they struggle to decide whether to take medications and, if so, which ones. Here are some of the research practices used by drug companies that compromise the credibility of their studies:

- Commissioning multiple studies to assess a drug's effectiveness and then reporting only on the research most flattering to their product.[16]
- Firing doctors who serve as well-paid consultants on effectiveness studies if they report negative findings. This puts pressure on doctors to search their data for positive results.[17]
- Hiring professional ghostwriters to pen favorable articles which are then published under the names of real doctors who are paid for their services.[18]
- Hiring different physician researchers to publish slightly different versions of the same set of complimentary findings in several journals to give the impression that much independent evidence points to the effectiveness of a particular drug.[19]
- Comparing their medication with others by giving control groups only the lowest effective dosage of the competing drug.[20]
- Devising questions to measure symptom relief in ways that maximize the likelihood of positive reports. They may use different measurement procedures when evaluating the effectiveness of competing drugs.[21]
- Failing to systematically ask study respondents about certain side effects, thus ensuring that rates of ad-

verse reactions are greatly minimized. Also, since doctors rarely report adverse effects to the FDA after a drug has appeared on the market, as they are expected to do, the reported rates of troublesome side effects are enormously underestimated.[22]

- Limiting drug trials to short periods of time (often only several weeks). Drug companies rarely do long-term studies to determine how large populations experience medications over time.[23]

Pharmaceutical companies have infiltrated every area of medical research, training, and practice, greatly undermining the credibility of medical knowledge in general. Continuing education programs for physicians are subsidized by pharmaceutical companies and dominated by speakers on their payrolls. Physicians are paid handsome bounties for each person they help to enroll in a company's drug study. Major hospitals, research centers, and universities now depend substantially on support from drug companies. Drug representatives lavish doctors with free samples, gifts, and dinners. The industry's lobby in Washington is larger than that for any other private interest.[24] Many researchers who publish findings in the most prestigious medical journals have financial ties to drug companies, as do many experts who sit on FDA panels deciding a drug's future. Such dispensing of "drug money" has created so many conflicts of interest that the quality of knowledge available to physicians, regulatory agencies, and patients has become tainted. Unholy alliances based on mutual financial interest produce junk science whose purpose is less the discovery of truth than the marketing of products.[25]

"Psychopharmacology," writes T. M. Luhrmann,

> is the great, silent dominatrix of contemporary psychiatry. It is what psychiatrists do that other mental health professionals cannot do; and as mental health jobs become defined more by their professional specificity, more and more psychiatrists spend more of their time prescribing medications. This is where the weight of most psychiatric research is placed. More money is spent developing, testing, and analyzing psychopharmacological drugs than in any other area of psychiatry; more people are involved in the research; more patients (these days) are probably touched by these agents than by anything else the psychiatric profession does.[26]

Moreover, experimental studies are often inconclusive. Rarely does the antidepressant medication far exceed the placebo in effectiveness, and sometimes subjects in the control group actually report greater symptom relief.[27] Equally important, the newer classes of antidepressant medications (the SSRIs), hyped as the latest wonder drugs, are actually no more effective than categories of medications (for example, tricyclic antidepressants) that were discovered in the late 1950s.[28] Finally, these studies have no way to assess whether medications work better than positive life changes. The sociologist Allan Horwitz asks:

> How does the effectiveness of the medication com-
> pare with entering a new career, joining a gym, going
> to religious confession, or returning to school?
> Would a disorder respond better to an entirely differ-
> ent kind of therapy than to medicine? Would people
> who suffer from distressing romantic relationships
> gain more from entering new relationships than from
> taking an anti-depressant? We cannot, of course, de-
> sign an experimental study that provides people with
> new romantic partners, so we don't know. But the
> finding that receiving a particular medication is supe-
> rior to not receiving this medication indicates noth-
> ing about the effectiveness of medication compared
> to alternatives such as changing social circumstances
> or providing other sorts of therapies.[29]

Socializing both patients and doctors to the idea that bothersome moods are biological diseases occurs on two fronts. First, all of us are instructed daily via drug adver- tisements that we need not put up with unpleasant and "abnormal" feelings when eradicating them is so easy.[30] Second, pharmaceutical companies sponsor drug semi- nars and employ a small army of salesmen to give doctors the tools that will make their patients happy. Most anti- depressants are prescribed by family physicians, whose knowledge of psychiatric medications is often limited to clinical experience, to what they are told by drug com- pany representatives, and to what they can learn in the *Physician's Desk Reference.*[31] Although doctors are often unsure about whether a patient's life circumstances or biology is causing his or her bad feelings, they largely fall back on biomedical discourse in deciding to dole out pills.

Given the vast numbers of people currently using psychotropic medications, it seems clear that Americans are increasingly giving medical pioneers freer access to their minds and feelings. We are rapidly moving closer to normalizing the idea that virtually any feelings short of complete happiness are unacceptable. A friend from New York told me that after she reported to her doctor that she had become "edgy and irritable" following September 11, he immediately suggested that she try Paxil. What does it say about the current state of medicine when healthy people experiencing appropriate emotions are routinely treated with powerful medications they do not really need?

I am certainly not arguing that medications be withheld from people whose illnesses have compromised their capacity to function in the world. I contend, rather, that doctors are practicing bad medicine when they ignore the Buddhist truth that life is difficult and hand out medications for the normal pains of daily living. The question is not whether to be respectful of people's pain and somehow attend to it. By contrast, we need to ask how we should conceptualize the vast middle range of emotional problems, what labels we should use in describing them, and what interventions are the most appropriate for minimizing them. If, in the end, the twin forces of pharmaceutical companies and psychiatric medicine take over the full continuum of uncomfortable human feelings, we will be that much closer to Huxley's "brave new world."

Consequences of Biological Psychiatry

Every person with whom I spoke had theories about the source of his or her difficulties. The great majority of interviewees attributed their bad, often crippling feelings to their immediate experiences as well as to their brain chemistry. Their ideas about the source of depressive illness rarely extended to the ways in which society is organized as a whole or to how broad cultural changes influenced their well-being. Alice was an exception. Could it be, as she suggested, that manic-depressive illness is most likely to arise in a manic society?

> I think that it's important to think about the way society . . . is constructing these diseases. Why has bipolar become so popular right now? What is it about this time and the culture that has brought this diagnosis out? I have a quick answer which is [that] there's great disparity in this country, and there's great inequalities, and I think there's tremendous motion. Things go very, very quickly now. You have 170 channels on TV, and kids can't sit still for more than ten minutes, and everything goes from, "It's wonderful, God Bless America," to people starving in our own streets, [and the government] sending people out to kill people. So in that way the disease, the illness . . . can become very socially constructed. . . . That's where I could say, "Maybe it doesn't even have to be biological. Maybe you don't even need the predisposition for it to manifest itself." So I think that's

> . . . how I see it. I don't see it as nature [or] nurture.
> Yes, both can play a part, but I'm more interested in
> how it is defined . . . through culture.

Indeed, why should we be surprised at the explosion of depressive illness in a society that increasingly separates us from social institutions and from one another? Why should we be surprised that up to 40 percent of unemployed women receiving welfare in order to care for their children at home screen positively for depression?[32] Why should we be surprised that increasing numbers of middle-class, white-collar workers are joining a new "anxious class" as corporations downsize and reengineer their companies, shipping jobs to places with better "business climates"?[33] Why should we be surprised that rates of depression are directly tied to social class in a society that "hyper-ghettoizes" poor people and cuts them off from the mainstream of society?[34] Why should we be surprised that among the best predictors of hospital admission for major mental illnesses is the state of the economy?[35]

The prevailing ideology in psychiatry privatizes human problems by seeking to change only the person's neurotransmitters. In this way, it is even more conservative than earlier attempts by psychiatry to reshape the patient's self through talk therapy so that the person might fit more comfortably into society. Neither approach recognizes that the solutions to human ills might best be accomplished by restructuring society itself.

Of course, we can see why healers might gravitate toward individualistic treatments of human pain. It is far easier to change individuals than it is to change ingrained social structures. Still, if we accept that factors such as poverty and gross inequality are deeply implicated in emotional illnesses, we must also accept that treatments focusing exclusively on brains are necessarily incomplete. More problematic still is the danger that disease metaphors will blunt our collective sensitivity to "structural" problems in society and thus our commitment to solving them.

The relentless medicalization of behaviors has bred a nation of victims. Given the ever-expanding list of behaviors over which we presumably have no control, nearly everyone these days can claim victim status of one sort or another. Should you draw the anger of family and friends by drinking too much, by craving too much sex, by maxing out your credit cards at shopping malls, by ignoring others in favor of time on the computer, or by threatening your health through food bingeing, you may claim an addiction. If you cannot control your anger, your abusive behavior toward family members, your inability to deal with authority, your anxiety at cocktail parties, or your failure to clean your house, you can find a doctor with both a diagnosis to explain things and medications to minimize the symptoms. Biology has become "the great moral loophole of our age."[36] This represents a remarkable transformation in a culture founded on an ethic of responsibility and the value of rugged individualism.

Traditional psychotherapy, with its emphasis on self-understanding, is directed at making patients *more responsible* for changing themselves and their behaviors. In contrast, biological psychiatry, with its lack of interest in the biographies of patients, teaches people to jettison the burden of responsibility. If psychiatry is itself of two minds about the question of responsibility, so also are patients and those close to them.[37] Through hundreds of interviews with emotionally ill people and their families, I have found that many are still ambivalent about questions of personal responsibility. They remain skeptical of the claim that everyone with a diagnosis of mental illness is hobbled by a brain disease completely beyond his or her control. Confusion persists about whether objectionable behaviors should be understood in terms of the illness or the person. Sufferers and caregivers must constantly navigate between the rhetoric of biological determinism and an expectation of personal responsibility.

This is not to say that mental illnesses cannot be utterly disabling. People suffering from major mental illnesses deserve parity of care with those suffering from illnesses that are more clearly physically based. Governments should address the needs of those whose conditions prevent them from full participation in the worlds of family and work. But I worry that the psychiatric trumpeting of brain diseases radically shifts the cultural conversation about our personal obligations to society. A "no-fault" culture will flourish to the degree that we buy into the idea of having greatly diminished control over our selves, our feelings, and our behaviors. As the ideas of biological psychiatry gain an even firmer hold on the culture, the imbalance between rights and responsibilities may become even more pronounced.[38]

Today Prozac is to antidepressants what Kleenex is to tissues. No book did more to awaken the public to a new generation of antidepressant medications than Peter Kramer's 1993 best-seller *Listening to Prozac.* Kramer previewed a world in which "what is constant in the self and what is mutable, what is necessary and what is contingent, would need . . . to be revised." All this was summed up in what Kramer famously termed "cosmetic psychopharmacology." He imagined a future of psychotropic medications so refined that we could choose whichever personality traits we wanted. Of course, it would be hard to distinguish honest free choice from the pressures to become the types of people favored by particular cultures. The book, in short, raises questions about self and social control:

> We have talked about medication as altering personality, taking a person with dysthymia and making her temperamentally hyperthymic, sunny, and social. This potential has disturbing overtones; it may lead us to imagine a future in which the culture at large considers the depressive personality to be illness and the hyperthymic type to be optimally healthy. It raises the possibility of taking a normal individual and reaching into his or her personality to alter a particular trait. . . . Here medication allows for tinkering with personality and particular mental styles. This possibility has worrisome implications, not only as regards the arrogance of doctors but as regards the subtly coercive power of social convention.[39]

It has been more than a decade since Kramer made his predictions, and perhaps we will yet see an age with psychiatric medications so finely calibrated that crafting precise changes to personality will be possible. Right now, though, as the stories throughout this book show, pills remain blunt and unpredictable instruments. Psychiatry's unbridled enthusiasm for and commitment to medications far exceed their actual effectiveness. However, the current gap between representation and reality does not diminish the legitimate concern expressed by Kramer that as biological psychiatry defines more and more human variation as abnormal, the presumed freedom of choice offered by ever-expanding pharmacopeias will only mask a process through which unacceptable diversity will be eliminated. The end result will be a reduction in human freedom through a homogenization of appropriate feelings and behaviors. Rather than celebrating human diversity, biological psychiatry circumscribes ever more tightly the range of allowable emotions and behaviors.

Whenever a society narrows its definition of acceptable human variation, the result is often greater oppression and illness. We see this clearly in the case of changing cultural standards of beauty. In medicine the very thin line between enhancement and therapy has blurred as plastic surgery has become more commercialized.[40] Once only a small proportion of people tampered with nature to "perfect" their bodies. Now plastic surgeons devote themselves to reconstituting millions of bodies through elective surgery. Though many people undoubtedly feel better after treatment, there is also a dark side to homogenizing breasts, bellies, and noses: It puts pressure on others to conform to narrowly constructed body standards, further devaluing those whose appearance is distant from the ideal. The connection between rigid cultural norms and illness production is dramatically evident in the arrival of anorexia nervosa and bulimia as historically new diseases with devastating consequences for a large number of people who, affected by a "cult of thinness," have pathologized their own perfectly normal bodies.[41]

One of the most widely debated psychiatric approaches to a newly minted disease is Ritalin therapy for children who are unable to sit still or pay sufficient attention to authority figures such as parents and teachers.[42] Critics worry that creeping definitions of disease are being applied to children whose behaviors may be troublesome but are hardly abnormal.[43] Once a new diagnosis is created, the number of people with the disease expands to include those whose behaviors simply do not conform to evolving standards. The terrain shifts subtly so that children formerly considered unconventional or deviant join the ranks of the sick. The social critic Francis Fukuyama draws a compelling analogy between Prozac and Ritalin as two drugs that "exchange one normal behavior in favor of another that someone thinks is socially preferable."

> There is a disconcerting symmetry between Prozac and Ritalin. The former is prescribed heavily for depressed women lacking in self-esteem; it gives them more of the alpha-male feeling that comes with high

serotonin levels. Ritalin, on the other hand, is prescribed largely for young boys who do not want to sit
still in class because nature never designed them to
behave that way. Together, the two sexes are gently
nudged toward that androgynous median personality, self-satisfied and socially compliant, that is the
current politically correct outcome in American
society.[44]

I remember reading a disturbing newspaper article on a
federally funded study designed to isolate the genetic basis for violent behavior. Researchers proudly spoke about
the relevance of their work for policy, noting that once
tests were able to reveal children with a biological predis-
position to violence, doctors could treat them with medications as a preventive measure. It frightens me that we
could be approaching an era of preemptive biology when
it seems reasonable to treat people for potential nonconformity on the basis of genetic correlations that are sub-
sequently termed diseases.[45] The medical historian David
Healy describes an evolutionary movement "from a the-
ocracy through democracy to a sanitocracy."[46] To be sure,
with each of biological psychiatry's successful incursions
into domains of feeling and personality, our appreciation
and tolerance for human variation diminishes. This is
deeply troubling given that democracy and freedom depend so heavily on respect for vastly different feelings,
opinions, and thoughts, and the liberty to challenge the
status quo via nonconformity.

*   *   *

To be wary of disease models of mental illness does not mean to dismiss biology's likely role in major depression, manic depression, and schizophrenia. There is danger in all single-minded models—biological or social—for explaining mental illness. Beginning in the 1960s, a number of sociologists and radical psychiatrists pushed a very good idea too far. They allowed the important notion that mental illness is socially constructed to morph into the idea that mental illness is a myth altogether.[47] Such social determinism is as foolish as the biological determinism I have been faulting. Allan Horwitz says it best when he notes that "while symptom constellations can be products of particular cultures . . . [this] does not mean that the underlying disorder is artificial. Because the particular symptoms . . . sufferers display are products of particular socio-cultural forces does not make their suffering any less real. For them, symptoms are not imaginary or simulated."[48]

The real challenge is to avoid dichotomous thinking. Positions that understand mental illness as solely a matter of nature or of nurture will always fall short. A healing discipline that frames human suffering only in terms of disease lacks commonsense validity. A bigger challenge, though, is to understand the economic, cultural, professional, and personal factors that foster false dichotomies in the first instance. By now, you should understand that my quarrel with psychiatry and pharmaceutical companies is not about drugs per se. I am far more bothered by the confluence of forces that lead doctors to *routinely* medicate for life distress. Indeed, "it seems hardly more advisable to treat minor ailments with psychiatric drugs than it is to shoot pheasants with elephant guns."[49]

No one, of course, can say exactly when normal distress becomes pathological pain. But if we are to err it should be on the side of not medicating the few who need it rather than medicating the many who do not need it. At the moment, such a conservative approach to medication is completely undermined by powerful social forces. It surely is bad medicine to alter the brains of those who suffer from the usual problems of living. Equally important, unwarranted medical intrusion into new frontiers of feelings, thoughts, and emotions potentially harms society. The more pills we dispense for normal distress, the more we avoid tackling our most difficult social problems, potentially undermine personal responsibility, and perhaps even threaten the sort of diversity necessary for a flourishing democracy.

Epilogue: Lessons from the Inside

When it comes to most complex life issues, people usually arrive at simple but profound truths largely through trial and error. Teenagers may not grasp the wisdom of their parents' admonitions until after they have done things their way. The daily realities of marriage carry little value for those caught up in a new romance. Any parent will tell you that no amount of observing and talking to others could have prepared them for life with children. Some adults spend years in therapy before absorbing what appear to be, from the outside, simple life lessons. In quite the same way, the conversations throughout this book suggest that internalizing basic ideas about medications may take years.

The purpose of this epilogue is to help people struggling with illness and medications to feel less alone in their plight. My grander hope is that the wisdom provided by those I interviewed will save others years of pain, confusion, and inadequate treatment.

Given the richness of experience conveyed in my interviews, it was not easy to distill all the knowledge expressed into a few principles. Still, when I asked interviewees what they wanted to pass along to readers, they agreed on seven suggestions: Ask for help early rather than trying to handle things on your own. Become an educated consumer right from the beginning. Recognize that drugs alone are not the answer. Have realistic expectations about medications. Move beyond the shame and stigma associated with mental illness. Appreciate what your illness can teach you about yourself and life in general. Don't give up hope.

Ask for Help

> *Don't try and do this on your own. It's way too big,*
> *way too hard. Ask for help. Be selective in who you ask*
> *for help, but ask for help. Get advice from other people.*
> *And give their advice a shot before you throw it out.*
> —unemployed woman, aged 47

Too often sage advice is born of regret. Many of the fifty interviewees told stories of going it alone for years before asking for help. They endured their pain to the point of desperation before seeking *anyone's* help. Many shared the experience of a middle-aged woman who explained: "Because of the time [that passed before] I sought help, I was really depressed. I wasn't moderately depressed. I was the stereotype that if you seek help you'll be judged differently by society forever." She made the case even more bluntly when she added: "[Ask] for help in the early moments and [don't wait] until it gets unmanageable. I used to tough it out and think that was virtuous. That was just stupid in hindsight."

In retrospect, interviewees saw stoic silence as ultimately self-defeating, for it only increased their pain. I heard many variations of these thoughts: "I just wish I had gotten help sooner." "I needed major help long before I got it." "There is help out there and you're not alone." "Character-building kinds of things just don't work." "You know, people say, 'Pick yourself up by your boot-straps.' There's no such thing as bootstraps. They don't work." Most people acknowledged that it is foolish to live with distress that clearly exceeds the normal pain of daily living. One man explained: "It was Confucius [who said], 'He who keeps doing the same thing expecting the results to change is a fool.' . . . [If] your tire is digging in and you're rolling back and forth in reverse and forward and you're still in the sand, then it's time to call a tow truck. And psychiatric meds might be a tow truck."

Another person made an interesting distinction between "normal unhappiness" and "neuro-unhappiness." The distinction suggests that at some point you need to acknowledge that your suffering is so persistent and deep that it goes well beyond the boundaries of life's usual ups and downs. Rather than relieving those who suffer from mental illness of responsibility, advocates of early intervention claim that people have an obligation to act on their own behalf (and, I might add, on behalf of those close to them). As one person warned: "Don't let the illness control your life. You have to control the ill-ness."

Become an Educated Consumer

> *Before taking any kind of psychiatric drug, know what you're taking. Ask questions. If the doctor doesn't do it*

> on [his or her] own, ask questions. Go to the library to
> research it. Go on the Internet. Whatever you have to
> do before you take that first pill, know what the possi-
> ble side effects are. Know if it's addicting. Educate
> yourself as best as you can. Talk to other people . . .
> who are taking it. Just don't pop a pill.
>
> —female market researcher, aged 35

By far the most consistent and clear advice I heard was about the necessity of maintaining autonomy in dealing with doctors and drugs. Here the advice is both to *question authority* and to *become an authority*. Adopting an active rather than a passive voice in managing illness is especially difficult during the early stages of treatment because "people go to doctors usually when they're feeling disempowered." Patients cannot afford to be compliant consumers. The first task is finding the right help. One woman stressed: "When you go to see a doctor, a psychiatrist, a psychologist, a social worker, [or] whatever . . . evaluate them and see them as a product that you are investing in. And because you see them as a product you're investing in, they deserve every bit of interrogation you can muster."

One young woman thought that shopping for doctors should be standard practice. Her advice was to interview at least three doctors before choosing one. The message from most people was to question authority:

> All of us trust our doctors much too much. . . . We
> need to remember that it's *our* lives.

I know plenty of people who will go to the doctor and the doctor will spend five minutes with them and say, "Take this," and they're like, "Okay." . . . I mean, God forbid!

If things are going okay and your doctor wants to change your medication, then they better have a damn good reason why.

If you're not happy with your doctor, don't stick with him. Negotiate with your doctor.

I've become much more actively involved in dialogue with this psychiatrist. . . . Back then they said, "Take this," [and] I took it.

A physician confirmed the validity of such advice:

One should advocate for oneself in a very strong way. If that means doctor shopping or if that means ranting to the human rights person at the hospital, [do it]! Don't ever sit back and just say this is it.

In order to have a constructive, two-way conversation with doctors, patients must become well informed about medications. Too many years of unquestioning compliance led many to stress the importance of educating oneself:

> Really research everything that you put into your
> body.

> Know what you are taking before you take it. . . . Just
> know what it can do to you and what the ramificat-
> ions can be.

> I think you really have to be more of an activist on
> your own behalf. You've got to do the research that a
> doctor just doesn't have the time to do.

> Understand that there are different drugs and there
> are pros and cons to [each one].

Equally important to satisfactory treatment is learning to
trust your own experiences with medications:

> You don't need somebody else to tell you this drug
> works for you because you know when it works for
> you and when it doesn't. And you shouldn't rely on
> someone to make the decision to take the drug or
> not to take the drug. . . . You're the only one who
> lives with you. You're the only one who feels what it
> feels like to take the drug.

One woman had, after much trial and error, learned
the art of what she called "open-minded vigilance." When
asked to share the most basic lesson she had learned over
the years, she replied:

> Maybe the message would have to do with . . . not be-
> ing too rigid. . . . I felt I needed to be open to medica-
> tion but . . . still somewhat skeptical. . . . So I had to
> be open in both directions, and I had to keep vigilant
> in both directions. So I guess I would say something
> like, "[Practice] open-minded vigilance."

Recognize That Drugs Are Not Enough

> *I want to say this for the recorder and for you. It is that
> it didn't take just a medication to make me better. It
> took the right therapist, the right medication, and the
> support group to get well. It's not just one thing.*
> —female health advocate, aged 57

These days it is hard to find insurance plans that will cover a combination of therapeutic approaches. Despite substantial evidence that talk and medication therapies work best in conjunction, treatment plans are largely driven by perceived economic exigencies. Because medications are viewed as a much cheaper response to mental health problems, they have clearly gained ascendancy as the most common treatment. Health bureaucracies and insurance companies have not caught up with what patients already know. The human and social costs of using pills alone are in the long run greater than the costs of a multifaceted approach to mental health. The experts who speak here recognize that their personal and family stability, their work productivity, and their ability to avoid costly hospitalizations are greatly increased when they receive a combination of talk and drug therapy.

Those taking psychotropic drugs for the first time should be mindful of what experience has taught others about how best to maximize emotional well-being:

> I have serious doubts about people who are on medication and not in therapy. . . . Medication is only part of it.

> Medication helps you reach that level of functioning so you can do things in psychotherapy.

> Drugs don't work by themselves and psychotherapy doesn't work by itself. . . . If you had drugs that made you feel better but you were not making a connection with someone else, you're gonna have a hard time.

> I feel so bad for people who really need both medication and counseling and they can't get the counseling . . . [or] won't stay with anyone very long.

> Drugs were just a piece of the puzzle. . . . If I had not done any of the other . . . work—emotionally, psychologically, spiritually, physically—I don't think I'd be out of pain.

> I don't think you can just sit back and take pills and say, "Well, eventually they'll kick in." I think you have to really work at it.

As the last two comments suggest, getting well is hard work. The notion that emotionally ill people need to explore multiple avenues leading to wellness is a welcome antidote to a passive patient model. By making people responsible for actively managing their own illnesses, this idea simultaneously restores their personal autonomy and diminishes the power of mental illness. There is wisdom in the following observation:

> I believe in this whole concept of recovery . . . and it's something that . . . requires work. . . . People with mental illness are not singled out for misery. I mean, other people have to struggle because they're poor, because they have to take insulin, because they get fired. . . . I don't want to belittle mental illness, but looking at it as a struggle like any other struggle takes away the enormity of it.

Sometimes therapeutic work consists of very small steps

> Keep moving.

> If you're able to get out and interact . . . your mental health is going to be better.

> Even when I get so down sometimes I have to . . . do one thing. Sometimes it is a walk, or just getting yourself out of bed, or drinking three glasses of water. . . . Do something that [requires] discipline.

> Routine has helped me when I've been depressed . . .
> daily prayer or whatever . . . to ground me.

That such small things can be seen as triumphs conveys the extraordinary courage and heroism associated with working toward greater wellness. One woman, a writer, described what reminded her of her own courage: "I read some of [my writing] aloud to my analyst. . . . Then you hear your spirit, you hear your courage coming back and you remember, 'This is who I am; this courageous person; this person who has achieved things, and this person with a very strong spirit.'"

Have Realistic Expectations

> *It's like people think they're going to take a pill and it's a happy pill, and then they're going to be happy. And really what it does is it balances out feelings. But it's a fairytale if people think they're going to take a pill and then run out in the street and say, "I'm happy." . . . That's not the way it is.*
>
> —female technical writer, aged 50

The accounts in this book converge on a difficult truth: Except in rare instances, medications do not cure affective disorders. Mental illnesses are chronic. There is typically an unpredictable ebb and flow to emotional distress. For some, difficult episodes of depression or mania are punctuated by periods of remission. Others describe good days and bad days. Yet others muddle along in a state of unrelenting sadness. Although most sufferers begin their explorations of medication with high hopes that pills will save them, they nearly always come to a more balanced and modest appraisal of what drugs can accomplish. Life might be easier if those new to medications began treatment with the consciousness of the depression-tested twenty-year-old who advised: "Don't have high expectations that this is going to be your cure-all and solve all your problems." Or the wisdom of another who explained: "The pills aren't my gods. . . . They're something I turn to because from forty years of experience [I know that] they will make me a little better." Having more realistic expectations does not devalue pills or diminish hope. However, new patients should know that their experiences will likely approximate that of the interviewee who told me: "Me on an SSRI is better than me not on an SSRI, [but] . . . I still get depressed. I still go through depression."

Novices to drug therapy should be apprised of another reality. Most of us expect that for every illness we bring to a physician there is a clear medication choice. Finding appropriate drugs to treat psychiatric symptoms, by contrast, often involves lengthy experimentation. Here's what my interviewees had to say:

> Expect an entire year to try different medications . . .
> until you feel better. . . . Many [other] medications
> you take for a period of time [and] you stop the med-
> ication. . . . Psychiatric conditions [don't] fit that

kind of model. . . . We have to get through our skulls
that it's a different situation.

There is a lot of fine-tuning that has to be done. . . .
You're going to have to adjust and adjust and adjust.

It's frustrating. . . . Believe me, I have thrown everything you can think of against the wall in my house
except my kitties. It's infuriating, but I don't know
what else to do.

Having realistic expectations should not dull a more
fundamental truth: for most people, patience pays off.
Despite the frustrations that accompany drawn-out trials
of different medications, most of the people I interviewed
believed that, on the whole, they were better off taking
the drugs: "I would say that medications really saved my
life." "Maybe no one is ever 100 percent sure that the medications are what is helping, but . . . I feel that way and
take the medications." In light of these experiences, perhaps the best advice is, "You gotta hang in there and give
[medications] a good chance."

Get Past the Shame

*Probably if it hadn't been for my son's illness and go-
ing to all those groups, I probably wouldn't have ever
reached the point where I would admit to almost anybody that I take medication. But you know, I do tell
people now, and I'm not ashamed of it. And actually*

> *we shouldn't be ashamed of it. But yeah, it took twenty*
> *years. It took me twenty years to reach that point.*
> —retired female office worker, aged 56

The instruction to let go of the shame attached to mental illness can be exceedingly hard to follow. Cultural attitudes are changing, but not nearly fast enough to insulate most sufferers from the stigma that multiplies the pain of mental illness. As the stories in this book have shown, most interviewees were extremely cautious in revealing their problems. At the same time, many of them successfully shed the self-blame that typically accompanies emotional illness. They speak best for themselves:

> I'm understanding more that the stigma is internal,
> that it's really not about somebody out there. It's re-
> ally about the way I think about myself.

> I would just like people to know that it is not a
> shameful thing; that even though I have felt shame,
> it's not a shameful thing.

I have learned from my conversations that the grip of shame is loosened when people internalize two fundamental beliefs. The first is "You are not your illness"; the second is "Your illness is not your fault."

I remember sitting in a support group one time and being struck by a comment at the beginning of the meeting. The meeting began with brief introductions during which nearly everyone said something like, "My name is

Joe and I'm a depressive." After all the introductions, a young woman suggested that it would be far better if people said, "Hello, my name is so and so and I suffer from depression." She wanted people to stop thinking about themselves exclusively in terms of their illness. There is great power in such a consciousness shift. The point is eloquently made by an interviewee who told me:

> Every time we take the medication it keeps constructing your identity as bipolar, or as whatever diagnosis, but you know, that is not who I am. It is something that I happen to have, like my mother had cancer. . . . It's not, in any way, the whole of me. It's a part of me. I am a teacher. I am a writer. I am a lover. I am a woman. [Mental illness] is just [something that] gets in the way a lot.

While earlier comments stress the belief that people with affective disorders need to work hard at becoming well, nearly everyone eventually came to the conclusion that they did not cause their illness:

> What you're thinking [during an episode] isn't you. It's the illness . . . and I've got to get help for these thoughts the way that you would get help for a cardiac arrest.

> The illness really has . . . biological symptoms . . . and [it is not] the person's fault. . . . They don't want to be ill.

I know that if I don't take my medications I'll get depressed. And that's not my fault. That's just something I have to contend with every day.

One comment captured best the interviewees' shared sentiments: "I am not responsible for being depressed. I can't help it. But I am responsible for what I choose to do with it." Of course, these thoughts cannot erase the opinions of the uninformed who stigmatize the mentally ill. But recognizing both that illness is only one part of who you are and that you did not cause it can help diminish the self-blame that only deepens the pain of depression.

Let Illness Be a Teacher

You feel like you have this window into truth when you're depressed. You see things that other people don't see.

—male peace activist, aged 22

Taking psychotropic drugs is one part of a powerful illness drama that inevitably transforms people. When I asked the people in my study what they had learned from their experiences, they often talked about the personal growth that resulted from their mental illness. There is, danger, of course, in emphasizing too strongly the positive aspects of a cruel illness. For example, by stressing the link between pain and creativity (as in discussions of van Gogh's genius or Sylvia Plath's poetry), we come dangerously close to romanticizing pain. Nonetheless, nearly everyone had stories about positive changes fostered by illness.

Though grateful for the relief provided by medications, some people noted that they had come to rely more on spiritual transformation than on medical cures:

> I'm a little amused by my pharmacologist. I can see how much more is . . . involved because this sort of illness is an illness of the spirit.

> I do meditation now and deep breathing to calm myself and center myself. And I try and put some structure into my day to manage some of the symptoms. And some of those things are helpful when the drugs aren't working.

> There was something so sublimely choreographed about my whole experience of illness that just kept pushing me toward confronting that vacuum in my life . . . to get back to the question of religion and spirituality.

> I heard a joke that religion is for people who don't want to go to hell, and spirituality is for people who have been there.

> You can view reality in . . . only two ways. It's either a torture chamber or a classroom. The data [are] consistent with both. [However], one way feels much better than the other.

Most people talked about seemingly small but profoundly humanizing changes. Several believed that their illness had deepened their empathy, sensitivity, and compassion. Others felt that the pain of illness had helped them focus on the moment. Sometimes this involved reorganizing their thinking in modest but personally meaningful ways:

> I've started to realize that some people who are very happy realize that life is not a great thing, but they don't let it control them. . . . I've started . . . being able to say, "Things are messed up, but what are you going to do?" I still want to go on and enjoy my breakfast. . . . Those eggs are still pretty good, so I'm going to smile about it.

For some people illness facilitated major practical changes. Several spoke of changing the way they approached their work:

> You work at a slower pace [and] you're less stressed. You're medicated [and] that's keeping you on an even keel. . . . So okay, I'm going to work at a pace that's good for me.

> I think part of my depression has to do with spending too much time working at a job . . . that I hardly even care about. . . . I've gone from working five days to three days and . . . that has been wonderful.

These people learned an important lesson in the face of a difficult illness: "Cut yourself some slack!" Others spoke directly to the importance of treating themselves well:

> One of the best things [my therapist] did for me was to give me permission to crash on some days.

> When I have a down day, I know perfectly well how to drop expectations to zero and not put any "shoulds" on myself at all. . . . And that practice stands me in good stead.

Everyone with whom I spoke certainly wished that their lives could be easier. At the same time, they acknowledged that their illnesses had influenced their views of the world and their sensibilities, shaping their identity in valuable ways.

Have Hope

> *The only way to survive it is to keep hopeful. As soon as you give in to despair, your journey becomes much blacker, uglier, and more painful.*
>
> —unemployed woman, aged 47

Sustaining hope can seem impossible to those suffering from depression, given that hopelessness is among the defining characteristics of the condition. At its worst, depression is so encompassing that each moment feels endless, and no matter how often one has been resurrected in the past, returning to life seems impossible this time. Here, for example, is a sampling of the ways people described the agony of depression: "I'd shake. I would feel gripped [in a way] that made it difficult to do anything—to think, to breathe." "I lost hope. . . . I was struggling. I was hanging on by a thread. I had thoughts of suicide." "I was basically just totally unable to function. I mean, I was in slow motion. . . . I could not get up in the morning. I couldn't sleep. . . . You feel like it's going to last forever. And there's not going to be any break." In fact, affective disorders are deadly. Half of those suffering from manic depression and 20 percent of those with major depression become hopeless enough to try suicide.

Still, as the stories in this book have shown, people do emerge from the deepest circles of emotional hell. Sometimes medication and therapy bring them back to life. Sometimes an episode simply runs it course. Sometimes the blackness of depression shades into a persistent, life-dulling gray. The most important thing to note is that large numbers of people do become well, or at least well enough that illness retreats into the background of their lives. I have always thought of the people I interview as heroic figures precisely because they keep looking forward even when life feels its bleakest. It takes great strength to try medication after medication when nothing seems to work.

The quotes I want to leave you with come from those who understand the importance of hope:

> I just thought nothing was going to work, but ultimately [a medication] lifted my spirits and things started to work out.

> Just don't give up . . . because the first [medication] isn't always going to be the right one.

> This business of drugs making such an amazing difference . . . that can happen and does happen.

> Don't give up. There is hope out there. There is support for everybody. Never give up.

On many occasions, people used precisely the same words to explain what they owed to medications: "They saved my life." One woman described just how deeply indebted she was to her therapist because "he truly taught me what hope was." When asked what he most wanted others to know, a middle-aged man immediately replied: "Number one is, don't give up the hope that things can turn out for the best with or without medication." When asked the same question, a long-time patient thought for a moment and said with intensity, "You *can* overcome suffering."

Appendix A

Getting Stories Straight

Despite a recent trend toward investigators' becoming a more integral part of the research process, scientific writing is largely equated with studies reporting on "objective" data gathered from large numbers of people.[1] For sociologists still hoping to build a cumulative science, large-scale survey research remains the prevailing model. Thus it is not surprising that many people continue to doubt the value of qualitative studies based on relatively few cases or interviews. Each time I write a book based on fifty or sixty interviews I expect the same questions and am never disappointed. I am always asked: "Can you really make any sort of generalizations from so few interviews? Just how did you secure your interviews? How do you know that people told you the truth about such a personal and sensitive issue as their mental illness?" In short, "How do you assess the validity of your data and analysis?"

Well-done qualitative studies bring human beings back into the research picture and, in so doing, have the potential to move readers profoundly. In a way that numbers rarely do, hearing people speak directly about the complexities of their lives allows readers to identify with them. The ultimate test of this study's validity will be that patients see themselves reflected in the stories told by others and understand their own situation more deeply as a result. Without question, the most exhilarating aspect of my work as a writer is hearing from readers who say they feel less alone after having read my work and have found new ways to think about their particular circumstances.

Many social scientists aspire to document fundamental truths about society. This may be a laudable goal, but I am not at all sure that it is the right one for the "social" sciences. While I feel obliged to collect data as carefully as possible, my mission in this book has not been to reveal a definitive truth about the experience of using psychiatric medications. There are consistencies and uniformities in even the most chaotic human experiences, but there is no unitary truth when it comes to momentous life events. My research begins with the supposition that social life is a very messy affair and that our most realistic goal is to provide novel ways to look at social phenomena. I am less interested in global generalizations about human behavior than in providing powerful, trenchant, and compelling frameworks for interpreting experiences that resist pat explanations. In-depth interviewing allows us to appreciate the dialectic of commonality and variability intrinsic to such complicated matters as psychotropic drug use.

Disclaiming the status of "hard" scientist does not entitle a researcher to methodological or conceptual sloppiness. The analyses I have offered throughout this work on such matters as authenticity, identity, and commitment would make no sense unless thoroughly grounded in the conversations I had with the fifty interviewees. My softer science is rooted in a commitment to let the world "speak back" to me.[2] Social scientists produce theories about every imaginable dimension of social life. Too often, though, those theories arrive full-blown from the heads of researchers only to be imposed on the data collected. The logic of my work, based on people's words, is instead to *discover* important ideas.[3] I aim to create as tight a fit as possible between the interviews I conduct and my analyses. Rather than seeing my data as providing definitive explanations, I understand my interviews as allowing glimpses into important life experiences. The biologist Richard Lewontin raises provocative questions about the proper subject matter of the social sciences, even asking, "How can there be a 'social science'?" He concludes:

> The answer, surely, is to be less ambitious and stop trying to make sociology into a natural science, although it is, indeed, the study of natural objects. There are many things in the world that we will never know and many things that we will never know exactly. Each domain of phenomena has its characteristic grain of knowability. Biology is not physics, because organisms are such complex physical objects, and sociology is not biology because human societies are made by self-conscious organisms. By pretending

to a kind of knowledge that it cannot achieve, social science can only engender the scorn of natural scientists and the cynicism of humanists.[4]

Given the goals of my writing, I resist strict numerical guidelines for evaluating the adequacy of my sample and analysis. Too often, small-sample interview studies like mine are viewed as informative, interesting, and sensitizing, but only as helpful adjuncts to the real work of social science. My bias is precisely the reverse. I begin my inquiry into an issue like psychiatric drug use and find that the bulk of the existing research consists of numbers describing the strength of various statistical relationships. Although certainly helpful, such research leaves out what is most important to me: I want to know about the struggles, emotions, hopes, and disappointments of real people. I find it dehumanizing to reduce dramatic, life-altering experiences to a series of indexes and causal models. Though I cannot claim that my sample of fifty people is necessarily representative of some larger population, I gladly trade breadth for depth.

I may not share exactly the same scientific goals as many of my colleagues, but I agree that we should all be mindful of the strengths and limitations of our claims. After all, I am writing as a sociologist rather than as a novelist, a poet, a journalist, or a memoirist. I am thereby implicitly claiming that there is something about the story I have told in this book that is, at the least, different from the ones that novelists, poets, journalists, or memoirists might tell about psychiatric drugs. I would not have bothered to spend hundreds of hours interviewing people unless I thought my work would lead to unique insights into the phenomenology of psychiatric drug use. That being so, I certainly have an obligation to consider the ways in which my findings might be an artifact of my sample and methods.

Although this book relies on fifty interviews focused explicitly on medications, my thinking has also been shaped by my prior research on depression. The fifty interviews I conducted for my book *Speaking of Sadness* inevitably touched on medication experiences, so it would not have made sense to disregard those materials. The fact that both sets of interviews converge on similar patient concerns about psychiatric drugs strengthens my faith in the patterns described throughout this book. As with the interviews conducted for *Speaking of Sadness,* the forty adults I interviewed for this book varied by sex (14 males, 26 females); age (under 20 = 3, 20s = 11, 30s = 3, 40s = 5, 50s = 17, 60 = 1); occupation (professionals = 14, white collar = 8, blue collar = 1, students = 9, unemployed = 4, retired = 4); educational achievement (high school = 4, college = 22, graduate education = 14); and marital status (married = 10, single, never married = 21, single, divorced = 6, single, widowed = 1, living together = 2).

Even if I wanted my sample to approximate the characteristics of all those who are treated with psychiatric drugs, there is no way to know precisely what that larger universe might look like. Fifty years ago we could safely say that nearly everyone who took psychiatric drugs was hospitalized with major depression or schizophrenia. By the 1970s, millions of essentially healthy Americans (especially housewives) were filling prescriptions for "minor" tranquilizers that, not incidentally, turned out to have major problems. Today, the newer classes of antidepressants are being used by a wide range of people—from those with chronic and debilitating mental illnesses requiring multiple hospitalizations to those wanting to feel even "better than well."[5] In contrast, everyone with whom I talked for this book had received an "official" diagnosis of depression or manic depression. Eighteen of the forty adults were seriously ill enough to have been hospitalized. Thus, while there is a range of illness experience among those sampled, the respondents for this study have been on the whole more seriously ill than would be a representative sample of Americans using the same medications.

Initially, I made contact with several interviewees through my connections at MDDA. Most of the people who attend the self-help meetings have experienced severe episodes of mental illness. To be certain that my sample was not unfairly skewed toward such very ill people, I recruited interviewees from other populations as well. I contacted therapists for referrals, sought volunteers from among my own students, and asked colleagues and friends to pass along the word that I wanted to interview people who were using psychiatric medications. Further, after each completed interview I encouraged the respondent to tell others about my study. In this way, my sample was ultimately drawn from a number of sources, ensuring that the stories I heard did not reflect only the experiences of a narrow population.

Far more challenging than recruiting adult interview-ees was the task of securing ten interviews with teenagers. Quite appropriately, the Institutional Review Board at Boston College has many safeguards in place to ensure that human subjects, especially vulnerable populations, are not harmed as a result of their participation in a research study. I could not approach young people directly because I first had to gain the approval of their parents or guardians. Here again, I largely relied on others who were regularly in contact with troubled teenagers and their parents or guardians. In one case I was directed to an organization called the Parents Professional Advocacy League. I agreed to give a keynote address at their annual dinner in exchange for help in contacting students and parents. I also sought the help of therapists who specialize in treating adolescents. Finally, I worked with administrators at an alternative high school for emotionally troubled teenagers. Both parents and children had to sign special consent forms before an interview could be arranged. It took many months of networking before I was finally able to record the conversations of a diverse group of teenagers. They came from different class backgrounds, attended both suburban and urban schools, and suffered from different illnesses.

Recruiting a range of interviewees is a daunting enough task. The more significant challenge, though, is to have conversations that get to the emotional core of people's illnesses and medication experiences. While I do not believe that conducting a good interview necessarily requires researchers to have had experiences similar to those of interviewees, my own drug and illness biography was plainly valuable in doing this research. Many emotionally ill people feel that others simply cannot comprehend their special pain. Not only did I make immediately plain my personal motives for doing the research, but I also occasionally used my own experiences as the basis for interview questions. These revelations contributed to the sort of trust and rapport that has to be established quickly in a one-shot conversation.

Interviewing teenagers was a real learning experience for me. Although I had constructed a special interview guide for my talks with them, their occasional blank stares reminded me that I was still talking too much like a professor. As the interviews progressed I learned to tone down my language. Students also quickly pointed out that my knowledge of teenage popular culture was hopelessly inadequate. It no doubt helped that I could laugh at myself. These slight problems aside, I think the teenagers leveled with me about their feelings. It mattered to them that I took pills myself and that I wanted to talk with them because *they* were the experts on teenage depression and medication use. As I learned from the content of their interviews, adults are too rarely respectful of what teenagers know and feel.

Instructing people on how to conduct a good in-depth interview is rather like giving hints on how to make engaging party conversation. For the conversation to flow smoothly, researchers must be deeply attentive to their respondents, have a sense about when to intervene in the conversation, when to follow up on unexpected comments, when to probe for more information about sensitive matters, when to commiserate with respondents, and when to steer the conversation in a new direction. Such things are not easily taught or learned.

In general, there was a predictable flow to the interviews. The first half-hour to forty-five minutes proceeded somewhat tentatively. I described the purposes of my work and began with unthreatening questions about age, occupation, religion, medical diagnosis, and the like. During the early part of the interview, individuals were no doubt assessing the worth of my study, their ease in talking with me, and, above all, my trustworthiness. The conversation often began in earnest after I asked the open-ended question, "When did it first enter your consciousness that something was *really* wrong?" For the next two hours or so, stories poured out. In many cases accounts were punctuated by strong emotions, often by tears. At the end of our time together, most respondents thanked *me* for the chance to articulate their experiences. Often, they said that my "sociological" questions provoked them to see aspects of their biographies differently.

Unlike survey research studies, in which analysis normally begins only after all the data have been collected, in-depth interview studies allow for the simultaneous collection and analysis of data. Qualitative researchers should attend to their interview transcripts as the research progresses, looking for emerging themes and plausible lines of analysis. Often ideas emerging from earlier interviews are incorporated into later ones, thus allowing the researcher to test preliminary hypotheses during the course of data collection. My own style is to write memos regularly about significant themes in the data. Some of the ideas in those memos hold up as new interviews are conducted, others are modified, and still others are discarded. Throughout, my goal is to remain as close to the data as possible so that my writing will be deeply embedded in the stories I hear.

As my vision for this book took shape, I divided the interview materials into several "data books" on such broad subjects as identity, significant others, and therapy. I spent months scouring these pages, making extensive marginal notations about repeating themes in the words of respondents. I continually asked, "What are the conceptual or analytical stories to be told from these materials?" For example, I became increasingly convinced that drug and romantic relationships share interesting similarities. Thus, the notion of "married to medication" took shape as an organizing device for Chapter 3. To be sure, there were other frameworks that could have been used for a chapter on commitment. The decision to exploit the marriage analogy was itself a kind of commitment to one plausible story line.

Each chapter in this book moved through a similar process. After conducting my interviews, I knew the fundamental direction that this book would take. At the same time, writing each chapter was a unique adventure filled with uncertainty and surprise. No matter how much I write, each article or book chapter begins with the same doubts: "Will I find a compelling way to pull together the interview materials? Will I be able to use the interviews in a fashion that will be both true to their substance and conceptually engaging?" Writing often moves in totally unanticipated directions as the story most worth relating becomes clear only in the telling. However, if you choose an important subject for study, have the interpersonal skills to be a good interviewer, live with your data, and have an extraordinary tolerance for ambiguity, you may very well bring new perspectives to important matters.

The story I wanted to tell in this appendix is that I am as much a craftsperson as a scientist.[6] In the end, no set of data speaks for itself. The logic of science does not itself produce interesting and powerful ideas. All that can be said about insight is that "to conceive fruitful original ideas, one must have talent, must immerse oneself in the available knowledge, and think very hard."[7] I have tried my best to respect the stories I heard and to think creatively about them. Ultimately, of course, it is up to you to decide whether I have sufficiently captured the respondents' experiences to teach you something new and valuable about psychiatric medications and identities.

Appendix B

Commonly Prescribed Drugs for Anxiety and Depression

U.S. BRAND NAME	GENERIC NAME	U.K. BRAND NAME
Adderall	amphetamine/ dextroamphetamine	Adderall
Ativan	lorazepam	Ativan
Aventyl, Pamelor	nortriptyline	Allegron, Aventyl
Benadryl, Hydramine, Benahist, Hydril, Sleep-eze, Sominex	diphenhydramine hydrochloride	Medinex, Sleepia, Nytol
BuSpar	buspirone	Buspar
Celexa	citalopram	Cipramil
Clozaril	clozapine	Clozaril
Depakote, Depakene, Dalpro	divalproex = valproic acid	Convulex
Desyrel, Trazon, Trialodine	trazodone	Molipaxin
Dexedrine	dextroamphetamine sulfate	Dexedrine
Effexor	venlafaxine	Effexor
Elavil, Endep, Emitrip	amitriptyline	Trytizol, Lentizol
Eskalith, Lithonate, Lithotabs, Lithobid, Cibalith	lithium carbonate, liskonum, priadel	Camcolit
Haldol	haloperidol	Dozic, Serenace
Janimine, Norfranil, Tofranil, Tipramine	imipramine	Tofranil
Klonopin	clonazepam	Rivotril

U.S. BRAND NAME	GENERIC NAME	U.K. BRAND NAME
Lexapro	escitalopram	Cipralex
Nardil	phenelzine	Nardil
Neurontin	gabapentin	Neurontin
Norpramin	desipramine	Pertofran
Paxil	paroxetine	Seroxat
Prozac	fluoxetine	Prozac
Remeron	mirtazapine	Zispin
Risperdal	risperidone	Risperdal
Ritalin	methylphenidate	Ritalin
Sinequan, Adapin, Zonalon	doxepin	Sinequan
Stelazine, Suprazine	trifluoperazine	Stelazine
Thorazine, Ormazine	chlorpromazine hydrochloride	Largactil
Topamax	topiramate	Topamax
Valium, Vazepam	diazepam, tensium, atensine	Valium, Rimapam
Wellbutrin	bupropion	(not available)
Xanax	alprazolam	Xanax
Zoloft	sertraline	Lustral
Zyprexa	olanzapine	Zyprexa

Notes

1. Giving Voice

1. The sample for this book consists of fifty interviews. Forty of the interviewees were eighteen years or older, and ten were children between the ages of thirteen and seventeen. The children's views are presented in Chapter 6.

2. See, for example, L. Slater, *Prozac Diary* (New York: Random House, 1998); K. Jamison, *An Unquiet Mind: A Memoir of Moods and Madness* (New York: Knopf, 1995); S. Kaysen, *Girl, Interrupted* (New York: Random House, 1993); S. Plath, *The Bell Jar* (New York: Bantam, 1972); N. Mairs, *Plaintext Essays* (Tucson, Ariz.: University of Arizona Press, 1986); W. Styron, *Darkness Visible: A Memoir of Madness* (New York: Random House, 1990); E. Wurtzel, *Prozac Nation* (Boston, Mass.: Houghton Mifflin Co., 1994).

3. S. Krieger, *Social Science and the Self* (New Brunswick, N.J.: Rutgers University Press, 1991), p. 4.

4. A. Kleinman, *The Illness Narratives* (New York: Basic Books, 1988), p. 8.

5. P. Kramer, *Listening to Prozac* (New York: Viking, 1993).

6. J. Davis-Berman and F. Pestello raise this and related questions about identity in their article "The Medicated Self," in N. Denzin, ed., *Studies in Symbolic Interaction: A Research Annual* (New York: Elsevier, 2005).

7. Slater, *Prozac Diary,* p. 49.

8. Ibid., p. 179.

9. P. Rieff, *Triumph of the Therapeutic* (New York: Harper and Row, 1966).

10. See C. Elliott, "Pursued by Happiness and Beaten Senseless: Prozac and the American Dream," in C. Elliott and T. Chambers, *Prozac as a Way of Life* (Chapel Hill, N.C.: University of North Carolina Press, 2004).

11. In Appendix A, "Getting Stories Straight," I explain my methodology in this study and consider the ways small-sample interview studies like mine can contribute more to our

understanding of issues like mental illness than can much larger statistical studies.

12. H. Koplewicz, *More Than Moody: Recognizing and Treating Adolescent Depression* (New York: The Berkley Publishing Group, 2002); S. Barondes, *Better Than Prozac: Creating the Next Generation of Psychiatric Drugs* (New York: Oxford University Press, 2003).

13. P. Breggin, *Toxic Psychiatry: Why Therapy, Empathy, and Love Must Replace the Drugs, Electroshock, and Biochemical Theories of the "New Psychiatry"* (New York: St. Martin's Press, 1991); *Brain-Disabling Treatments in Psychiatry: Drugs, Electroshock, and the Role of the FDA* (New York: Springer, 1997); *Psychiatric Drugs, Hazards to the Brain* (New York: Springer, 1983); *Talking Back to Prozac: What Doctors Won't Tell You about Today's Most Controversial Drug* (with Ginger Ross Breggin) (New York: St. Martin's Press, 1994); *Your Drug May Be Your Problem: How and Why to Stop Taking Psychiatric Drugs* (with David Cohen) (Reading, Mass.: Perseus Books, 1999). See also T. Szasz, *Ideology and Insanity* (Garden City, N.Y.: Anchor Books, 1970); R. Laing, *The Politics of Experience* (New York: Ballantine Books, 1967); E. Goffman, *Asylums: Essays on the Social Situations of Mental Patients* (Garden City, N.Y.: Doubleday Anchor, 1961).

2. Unwelcome Careers

1. A. Solomon, *The Noonday Demon: An Atlas of Depression* (New York: Scribner's, 2001); S. Nolen-Hoeksema, *Sex Differences in Depression* (Stanford, Calif.: Stanford University Press, 1990); D. Jack, *Silencing the Self: Women and Depression* (Cambridge, Mass.: Harvard University Press, 1991); See also R. Simon, "Revisiting the Relationships among Gender, Marital Status, and Mental Health," *American Journal of Sociology* 107 (January 2002): 1065–1096.

2. Jack, *Silencing the Self.*

3. See A. Hochschild, *The Managed Heart: Commercialization of Human Feeling,* 20th anniversary ed. (Berkeley, Calif.: University of California Press, 2003).

4. K. Jamison, *An Unquiet Mind: A Memoir of Moods and Madness* (New York: Knopf, 1995), 89.

5. See, for example, P. Conrad, "The Meanings of Medication: Another Look at Compliance," *Social Science and Medicine* 20 (1985): 29–37; S. Winnick et al., "How Do You Improve Com-

pliance?" *Pediatrics* 115 (2005): 718–724; P. Weiden and N. Rao, "Teaching Medical Compliance to Psychiatric Residents: Placing an Orphan Topic into a Training Curriculum," *Academic Psychiatry* 29 (May–June 2005): 203–210; N. Kerse et al., "Physician-Patient Relationship and Medical Compliance: A Primary Care Investigation," *Annals of Family Medicine* 2 (September–October 2004): 455–461.

6. See K. Charmaz, *Good Days, Bad Days* (New Brunswick, N.J.: Rutgers University Press, 1991).

7. Psychiatrists use the term "treatment resistant" to describe patients who do not improve with medication. Interestingly, those who do not respond to antidepressant medications are said to suffer from "atypical" depression.

8. Tricyclic antidepressant medications were developed in the 1950s and 1960s. Because they affect multiple neurotransmitters in the brain, they are thought to have more side effects than the newer class of SSRIs, which target the specific neurotransmitter serotonin.

9. Allan Horwitz, *Creating Mental Illness* (Chicago: University of Chicago Press, 2002).

10. MAOIs work by inhibiting a brain enzyme called monoamine oxidase. Patients taking MAOIs must avoid a substantial list of foods that can interact with the medication and cause dangerously high blood pressure.

11. Benzodiazepines comprise a category of drugs that include Ativan, Klonopin, Valium, and Xanax. Though initially effective in reducing anxiety, these medications can become addictive. It is generally advised that people use benzodiazepines to interrupt dramatic episodes of anxiety, such as a panic reaction, but that these medications not be used over extended periods of time.

12. The degree to which people may experience withdrawal is related to a drug's half-life. The shorter the half-life, the faster it leaves a person's system, and the more likely the person is to experience withdrawal systems when stopping the medication.

13. Atypical antidepressants such as Wellbutrin simultaneously target the neurotransmitters dopamine and norepinephrine.

14. The claim, largely supported by the drug industry, that antidepressants are effective 80 percent of the time is questionable since the word "effective" is so vague. Most people

equate effectiveness with a resolution of the problem, so to include in the 80 percent figure all those who report *any* degree of relief is misleading.

15. E. Becker, *The Denial of Death* (New York: Free Press Paperbacks, 1997).

16. Ibid., p. 26.

17. The diagnosis "generalized anxiety disorder, not otherwise specified" refers to a "free-floating" state of anxiety that is not firmly bounded. For example, a person with a diagnosis of generalized anxiety would be differentiated from someone who suffers specifically from panic disorders or from another particular phobia.

18. D. Karp, *Speaking of Sadness: Depression, Disconnection, and the Meanings of Illness* (New York: Oxford University Press, 2000).

3. Married to Medication

1. H. Blumer, *Symbolic Interactionism: Perspective and Method* (Englewood Cliffs, N.J.: Prentice Hall, 1969).

2. P. Berger and H. Kellner, "Marriage and the Social Construction of Reality," in P. Berger, ed., *Facing up to Modernity* (New York: Basic Books, 1977). See also P. Berger and T. Luckmann, *The Social Construction of Reality* (Garden City, N.Y.: Doubleday, 1967).

3. H. Becker, "Notes on the Concept of Commitment," *American Journal of Sociology* 66 (1960): 32–40.

4. P. Kramer, *Should You Leave?* (New York: Scribner's, 1997).

5. R. Findling, *The Commitment Cure: What to Do When You Fall for an Ambivalent Man* (Avon, Mass.: Adams Media, 2004). The self-help section of bookstores is filled with books on commitment phobia. It is, though, interesting to note that the emphasis of these books is on the greater difficulties that women have in getting men to commit than vice versa.

4. Searching for Authenticity

1. See J. Gamson, *Claims to Fame: Celebrity in Contemporary America* (Berkeley, Calif.: University of California Press, 1994).

2. See, for example, C. Taylor, *The Ethics of Authenticity* (Cambridge, Mass.: Harvard University Press, 1991); C. Elliott and T. Chambers, eds., *Prozac as a Way of Life* (Chapel Hill, N.C.: University of North Carolina Press, 2004); C. Elliott, *Better*

Than Well: American Medicine Meets the American Dream (New York: W. W. Norton, 2003).

3. C. Elliott, *Better Than Well,* p. 26.

4. Erving Goffman devoted his academic life to exploring the intersection of self and society. Goffman's model of interaction came to be known as a "dramaturgical" model since he maintained that human beings were performers who were consciously constructing self-images and impressions in order to elicit desirable responses from different audiences. Among his many books that play out the stage metaphor are *The Presentation of Self in Everyday Life* (New York: Doubleday Anchor, 1959); *Behavior in Public Places* (New York: Free Press, 1963); *Stigma: Notes on the Management of Spoiled Identity* (Englewood Cliffs, N.J.: Prentice Hall, 1963); *Interaction Ritual* (New York: Doubleday Anchor, 1967); *Strategic Interaction* (Philadelphia: University of Pennsylvania Press, 1969).

5. See R. Bellah et al., *Habits of the Heart: Individualism and Commitment in American Life* (Berkeley: University of California Press, 1985); A. Etzioni, *The Essential Communitarian Reader* (Lanham, Md.: Rowman and Littlefield Publishers, 1998).

6. A primary theme of the sociological literature on emotions is that people who are properly socialized are able to show the appropriate emotions called for in a given social situation and to avoid expressions of inappropriate emotions. For example, people who laugh during a funeral might be thought deviant because the situation calls for a display of grief whether or not one genuinely feels it. For a sociological perspective on emotions see A. Hochschild, "Emotion Work, Feeling Rules, and Social Structure," *American Journal of Sociology* 85 (1979): 551–575; A. Hochschild, *The Managed Heart: Commercialization of Human Feeling,* 20th anniversary ed. (Berkeley, Calif.: University of California Press, 2003); J. Barbalet, ed., *Emotions and Sociology* (Malden, Mass.: Blackwell, 2002); J. Turner and J. Stets, *The Sociology of Emotions* (New York: Cambridge University Press, 2005).

7. K. Jamison, *An Unquiet Mind: A Memoir of Moods and Madness* (New York: Knopf, 1995), pp. 91–92.

8. See J. Clair, D. Karp, and W. Yoels, *Experiencing the Life Cycle: A Social Psychology of Aging* (Springfield, Ill.: Charles Thomas Publishers, 1993).

9. Perhaps more than ever, women today are "victimized" by cultural standards of thinness. It is hard to think of a personal attribute more connected to self-esteem than weight. Sharlene Hesse-Biber has explored these matters in *Am I Thin Enough Yet? The Cult of Thinness and the Commercialization of Identity* (New York: Oxford University Press, 1996).

10. The much higher percentage has been reported to me in several private conversations with clinicians.

11. D. Karp, *The Burden of Sympathy: How Families Cope with Mental Illness* (New York: Oxford University Press, 2001).

12. M. Kundera, *The Unbearable Lightness of Being* (New York: HarperPerennial, 1984), p. 8.

5. Significant Others

1. Pain and suffering are subjective experiences, and caregivers and others may begin to doubt the veracity of someone's complaints over time. This is especially true for those illnesses where there is no external evidence of the problem. Caregivers to the mentally ill are often confused about whether another's objectionable behaviors are actually caused by their illness. They may come to believe that the person in their care is taking advantage of the "sick role." See D. Karp, *The Burden of Sympathy* (New York: Oxford University Press, 2001), and T. Parsons, *Essays in Sociological Theory* (Glencoe, Ill.: Free Press, 1954). A caregiver's failure to believe that someone is suffering from a "real illness" is greatest for problems such as chronic fatigue syndrome and environmental illness, which are currently "contested illnesses," themselves a source of professional confusion. See S. Kroll-Smith and H. Floyd, *Bodies in Protest* (New York: New York University Press, 1997). For a more general analysis of the "economy of sympathy" in relationships see C. Clark, *Misery and Company: Sympathy in Everyday Life* (Chicago: University of Chicago Press, 1997).

2. The conventional therapeutic wisdom is that many emotional problems suffered by women are a consequence of their overdependence on relationships. Consequently, one purpose of therapy should be to help women become more independent. In their contrarian analysis, Jean Baker Miller and Irene Stiver maintain that such a perspective reflects a male-oriented view of human relationships. In fact, they ar-

gue, deep connections between people are healing. Consequently, they advocate a version of psychotherapy in which therapists and patients form deep bonds. See J. Miller and I. Stiver, *The Healing Connection: How Women Form Relationships in Therapy and in Life* (Boston: Beacon Press, 1997).

3. Perhaps the most famous study on the relationship between authority and obedience was conducted by Stanley Milgram. See S. Milgram, *Obedience to Authority: An Experimental View* (New York: Harper and Row, 1974).

4. Perhaps the most extensive cross-cultural research on the variability of meanings attached to the idea of mental illness has been accomplished by Arthur Kleinman and his colleagues. See, for example, A. Kleinman, *Rethinking Psychiatry: From Cultural Category to Personal Experience* (New York: Free Press, 1988); A. Kleinman and B. Good, eds., *Culture and Depression: Studies in the Anthropology and Cross-Cultural Psychiatry of Affect and Disorder* (Berkeley: University of California Press, 1985).

5. See M. Zborowski, "Cultural Components in Responses to Pain," *Journal of Social Issues* 8 (1953): 16–31; C. Edwards, R. Fillingim, and F. Keefe, "Race, Ethnicity, and Pain," *Pain* 94 (2001): 133–137.

6. A series of studies demonstrates a synergistic effect between drug therapies and psychodynamic talk therapies. The effectiveness of each form of therapy used independently is less than their combined use in the case of major depression. See A. Solomon, *The Noonday Demon: An Atlas of Depression* (New York: Scribner's, 2001); E. Good, "Chronic Depression Study Backs the Pairing of Therapy and Drugs," *New York Times* (May 18, 2000); L. Altshuler et al., "Treatment of Depression in Women: A Summary of the Expert Consensus Guidelines," *Journal of Psychiatric Practice* 7 (May 2001): 185–208.

7. Kleinman, *Rethinking Psychiatry,* p. 11.

8. Ibid., pp. 111, 137.

9. Ibid., p. 112.

10. Ibid., p. 140.

11. For a discussion of the present state of psychotherapy see T. M. Luhrmann, *Of Two Minds: The Growing Disorder in American Psychiatry* (New York: Knopf, 2000).

12. See Arthur Kleinman, *The Illness Narratives: Suffering, Healing, and the Human Condition* (New York: Basic Books, 1988); Klein-

man, *Rethinking Psychiatry;* Luhrmann, *Of Two Minds;* P. Baker, W. Yoels, and J. Clair, "Emotional Expression during Medical Encounters: Social Dis-ease and the Medical Gaze," in V. James and J. Gabe, eds., *Health and the Sociology of Emotions* (Oxford: Blackwell Publishers, 1996); J. Kronenfeld, "New Trends in the Doctor-Patient Relationship: Impacts of Managed Care on the Growth of a Consumer Protections Model," *Sociological Spectrum* 21 (2001): 297–317; D. Roter et al., "Communication Patterns of Primary Care Physicians," *Journal of the American Medical Association* 227 (1997): 350–356.

13. W. Yoels and J. Clair, "Never Enough Time: How Medical Residents Manage a Scarce Resource," *Journal of Contemporary Ethnography* 23 (1994): 185–213.

14. See Lauren Slater's essay on the dilemma posed for women who become pregnant while taking antidepressant medications. "Noontime," in N. Casey, ed., *Unholy Ghost: Writers on Depression* (New York: William Morrow, 2001).

15. See Karp, *The Burden of Sympathy.*

16. One study demonstrates how doctor-patient interaction changes when there is a third person in the examining room. See P. Baker, W. Yoels, and J. Clair, "Laughter in Triadic Geriatric Encounters: A Transcript-Based Analysis," in R. Erickson and B. Cuthbertson-Johnson, eds., *Social Perspectives on Emotions* (Greenwich, Conn.: JAI Press, 1997).

17. P. Berger and H. Kellner, "Marriage and the Social Construction of Reality," in Peter L. Berger, ed., *Facing up to Modernity* (New York: Basic Books, 1977).

6. Teens Talk

1. T. Hine, *The Rise and Fall of the American Teenager* (New York: HarperCollins, 1999), p. 2.

2. D. Karp, L. Holmstrom, and P. Gray, "Leaving Home for College: Expectations for Selective Reconstruction of Self," *Symbolic Interaction* 21 (1998), p. 255.

3. The ten interviews I conducted with students between the ages of thirteen and seventeen provide the core materials for this chapter. Several of the interviewees for this book were college students whose experiences with medications began during high school or earlier. Since their accounts often contained rich detail about their middle school and high school

years, I have used those interviews to supplement the materials gathered specifically for this chapter.

4. In his well-known book *Asylums: Essays on the Social Situations of Mental Patients* (Garden City, N.Y.: Doubleday Anchor, 1961), Erving Goffman describes how patients in a psychiatric hospital create an "underlife" within the institution. In addition to the formal structure of the hospital, composed of official rules and regulations, there is a separate world of informal rules and regulations (the underlife) created by the patients themselves. Goffman maintains that an underlife will emerge in any institution in which people's identities are muted or altogether stripped from them by those in power.

5. See L. Holmstrom, D. Karp, and P. Gray, "Why Laundry, Not Hegel? Social Class, the Transition to College, and Pathways to Adulthood," *Symbolic Interaction* 24 (2002): 437–462; D. Karp et al., "Leaving Home for College."

6. Raves are dance parties populated by teenagers. Teens have described them to me as stress-free events in which young people can exuberantly express themselves through dance. Raves are often associated with recreational drug use.

7. This finding was reported in M. Milner, *Freaks, Geeks, and Cool Kids: American Teenagers, Schools, and the Culture of Consumption* (New York: Routledge, 2004).

8. Ibid., p. 25.

9. See B. Ehrenreich, *Fear of Falling: The Inner Life of the Middle Class* (New York: Perennial Library, 1990).

10. See M. Danesi, *My Son Is an Alien: A Cultural Portrait of Today's Youth* (Lanham, Md.: Rowman and Littlefield, 2003), p. 40.

11. The term "public degradation ceremony" was used by H. Garfinkel in his book *Studies in Ethnomethodology* (Englewood Cliffs, N.J.: Prentice Hall, 1967).

12. See, for example, R. Sennett and J. Cobb, *The Hidden Injuries of Class* (New York: Norton, 1993).

13. R. Emerson and S. Messenger, "The Micro-Politics of Trouble," *Social Problems* 25 (1977), p. 122.

14. See E. Goffman, *Stigma: Notes on the Management of Spoiled Identity* (Englewood Cliffs, N.J.: Prentice Hall, 1963).

15. For examples of how members of stigmatized groups manage their identities see A. Roschelle and P. Kauffman, "Fit-

ting in and Fighting Back: Stigma Management Strategies among Homeless Kids," *Symbolic Interaction* 27 (Winter 2004): 23–46; W. Thompson, J. Harred, and B. Burks, "Managing the Stigma of Topless Dancing: A Decade Later," *Deviant Behavior* 24 (November–December 2003): 551–570; A. Nack, "Damaged Goods: Women Managing the Stigma of STDs," *Deviant Behavior* 21 (March–April 2000): 95–121; D. Waskul and P. Van der Riet, "The Abject Embodiment of Cancer Patients: Dignity, Selfhood, and the Grotesque Body," *Symbolic Interaction* 25 (2002): 487–513. On managing the stigma of mental illness, see S. Onken and E. Slaten, "Disability Identity Formation and Affirmation: The Experiences of Persons with Severe Mental Illness," *Sociological Practice* 2 (June 2000): 99–111; E. Wright, W. Gronfein, and T. Owens, "Deinstitutionalization, Social Rejection, and the Self-Esteem of Former Mental Patients," *Journal of Health and Social Behavior* 41 (March 2000): 68–90.

16. See S. Hesse-Biber, *Am I Thin Enough Yet? The Cult of Thinness and the Commercialization of Identity* (New York: Oxford University Press, 1996).

17. Max Weber's analysis of power and authority remains a sociological classic. For an overview of Weber's writings see H. Gerth and C. W. Mills, eds., *From Max Weber: Essays in Sociological Theory* (New York: Oxford University Press, 1958).

18. J. D. Salinger, *The Catcher in the Rye* (Boston: Little Brown, 1951).

19. Ibid., pp. 20–21. For an interesting treatment of this theme see T. Hine, *The Rise and Fall of the American Teenager* (New York: Bard, 1999).

7. High on Drugs

1. I am using the word "paradigm" in this context in a way that corresponds to Thomas Kuhn's well-known discussion of paradigm shifts in science. Kuhn's analysis appears in his book *The Structure of Scientific Revolutions* (Chicago, Ill.: University of Chicago Press, 1996).

2. See A. Horwitz and T. Scheid, eds., *A Handbook for the Study of Mental Health: Social Contexts, Theories, and Systems* (Cambridge, England: Cambridge University Press, 1999).

3. Ibid.

4. T. M. Luhrmann, *Of Two Minds: The Growing Disorder in American Psychiatry* (New York: Knopf, 2000), p. 266.

5. Ibid., p. 137.

6. P. Conrad and J. Schneider, *Deviance and Medicalization* (Philadelphia: Temple University Press, 1992).

7. See L. Slater, "Kafka's Boys: A Story of Sex and Serotonin," in C. Elliott and T. Chambers, eds., *Prozac as a Way of Life* (Chapel Hill, N.C.: University of North Carolina Press, 2004); H. Shaffer, M. Hall, and J. Vander Bilt, "'Computer Addiction': A Critical Consideration," *American Journal of Orthopsychiatry* 70 (April 2000): 162–168. For an analysis of how children are inducted into America's consumer culture, see J. Schorr, *Born to Buy: The Commercialized Child and the New Consumer Culture* (New York: Scribner's, 2004).

8. American Psychiatric Association, *Diagnostic and Statistical Manual of Mental Disorders,* 4th ed. (Washington, D.C.: American Psychiatric Association, 1994).

9. These numbers appear in C. Malacrida, *Cold Comfort: Mothers, Professionals, and Attention Deficit Disorder* (Toronto: University of Toronto Press, 2003), p. 25.

10. See, for example, E. Valenstein, *Blaming the Brain: The Truth about Drugs and Mental Illness* (New York: Free Press, 1998); D. Healy, *The Anti-Depressant Era* (Cambridge, Mass.: Harvard University Press, 1997); D. Healy, *The Creation of Psychopharmacology* (Cambridge, Mass.: Harvard University Press, 2002); S. Kirk and H. Kutchins, *The Selling of DSM: The Rhetoric of Science in Psychiatry* (New York: A. de Gruyter, 1992); P. Caplan, *They Say You're Crazy: How the World's Most Powerful Psychiatrists Decide Who's Normal* (Reading, Mass.: Addison-Wesley, 1995).

11. T. Szasz, *Pharmacracy: Medicine and Politics in America* (Westport, Conn.: Praeger, 2001), p. 29.

12. See J. Abramson, *Overdosed: The Broken Promise of American Medicine* (New York: HarperCollins, 2004), p. 117.

13. See J. Cohen, *Overdose: The Case against the Drug Companies* (New York: Penguin Putnam, 2001), p. 36.

14. See J. Magno et al., "Psychotropic Practice Patterns for Youth: A Ten-Year Perspective," *Archives of Pediatric Adolescent Medicine* 157 (2003): 17–25.

15. See, for example, S. Fried, *Bitter Pills: Inside the Hazardous*

World of Legal Drugs (New York: Bantam Books, 1998); Healy, *The Creation of Pharmacology;* D. Healy, *Let Them Eat Prozac: The Unhealthy Relationship between the Pharmaceutical Industry and Depression* (New York: New York University Press, 2004); K. Greider, *The Big Fix: How the Pharmaceutical Industry Rips Off American Consumers* (New York: PublicAffairs, 2003); M. Angell, *The Truth about Drug Companies* (New York: Random House, 2004).

16. Healy, *The Creation of Pharmacology,* p. 311.

17. Cohen, *Overdose,* pp. 135–137; Valenstein, *Blaming the Brain* p. 189.

18. Healy, *The Creation of Pharmacology,* p. 311; Cohen, *Overdose,* pp. 131–142.

19. Healy, *The Creation of Pharmacology,* p. 311; Cohen, *Overdose,* p. 141.

20. Cohen, *Overdose,* p. 135.

21. Ibid.

22. Fried, *Bitter Pills,* p. 64.

23. Valenstein, *Blaming the Brain,* p. 188.

24. Angell, *The Truth about Drug Companies,* p. 198.

25. The range of conflicts of interest that compromise health knowledge and treatment are detailed in J. Kassirer, *On the Take: How Medicine's Complicity with Big Business Can Endanger Your Health* (New York: Oxford University Press, 2005). Other researchers have detailed the way that financial conflicts of interest impact knowledge and social policy in a range of health domains. See, for example, E. Boyd, S. Lipton, and L. Bero, "Implementation of Financial Disclosure Policies to Manage Conflicts of Interest," *Health Affairs* 23 (2004): 206–214; J. White and L. Bero, "Public Health under Attack: The American Stop Smoking Intervention Study (ASSIST) and the Tobacco Industry," *American Journal of Public Health* 94 (2004): 240–250; E. Boyd, M. Cho, and L. Bero, "Financial Conflict of Interest Policies in Clinical Research: Issues for Clinical Investigators," *Academic Medicine* 78 (2003): 769–774; A. Wazana, "Physicians and the Pharmaceutical Industry: Is a Gift Ever Just a Gift?" *Journal of the American Medical Association* 283 (2000): 373–380. Although conflicts of interest create problems for physicians attempting to evaluate medical knowledge, efforts have been made to educate doctors about the methodological criteria best used to distinguish between

flawed and valid claims to knowledge. See G. Guyatt and D. Rennie, eds., *User's Guide to Medical Literature: Essentials of Evidence-Based Clinical Practice* (Chicago: AMA Press, 2002).

26. Luhrmann, *Of Two Minds,* p. 47.

27. Healy, *The Creation of Pharmacology,* p. 308.

28. Healy, *Let Them Eat Prozac,* p. 38.

29. A. Horwitz, *Creating Mental Illness* (Chicago, Ill.: The University of Chicago Press, 2002), p. 192.

30. For a variety of reasons, including direct advertising to consumers, patients are sometimes unsettled when doctors do not prescribe any medication for their symptoms. Patients expect to receive prescriptions, and this puts pressure on doctors to give them pills that, in the doctors' judgment, are not necessary. A good example of this practice is the prescription of antibiotic medications for viruses when doctors know that they will be of absolutely no medical use. There has been a good deal of debate about the nature and effects of drug advertising. See, for example, A. Holmer, "Direct-to-Consumer Advertising: Strengthening Our Health Care System, *New England Journal of Medicine* (February 14, 2002): 526–528; J. A. Nikelly, "Drug Advertisements and the Medicalization of Unipolar Depression in Women," *Health Care for Women International* 16 (1995): 229–242; Angell, *The Truth about Drug Companies,* pp. 123–126.

31. The *Physician's Desk Reference* is a comprehensive book that provides doctors with information about the uses and side effects of all FDA-approved medications. Often the entries for medications are based on the documents provided by drug companies on their own products.

32. T. Maher, "The Withering of Community Life and the Growth of Emotional Disorders," *Journal of Sociology and Social Welfare* 19 (1992): 125–143.

33. C. Derber, *Hidden Power: What You Need to Know to Save Our Democracy* (San Francisco: Berrett-Koehler, 2005).

34. See, for example, W. Eaton and C. Muntaner, "Socioeconomic Stratification and Mental Disorders," in A. Horwitz and T. Scheid, eds., *A Handbook for the Study of Mental Health* (Cambridge, England: Cambridge University Press, 1999). The term "hyper-ghettoization" comes from W. Wilson, *The Truly Disadvantaged: The Inner City, the Underclass, and Public Policy* (Chicago: University of Chicago Press, 1990).

35. M. Brenner, *Mental Illness and the Economy* (Cambridge, Mass.: Harvard University Press, 1973). See also M. Lennon, "Work and Unemployment as Stressor," in Horwitz and Scheid, *Handbook for the Study of Mental Health.*

36. Luhrmann, *Of Two Minds,* p. 8.

37. Ibid.

38. The sociologist Amitai Etzioni has written widely on the breakdown of community and the increasing imbalance between rights and responsibilities in the United States. See A. Etzioni, *The Spirit of Community* (New York: Simon and Schuster, 1993), and *The Essential Communitarian Reader* (Lanham, Md.: Rowman and Littlefield Publishers, 1998).

39. P. Kramer, *Listening to Prozac* (New York: Penguin Books, 1993), pp. 21, 249. See also Kramer's latest book, entitled *Against Depression* (New York: Viking, 2005), in which he details the destructive effects of depression on the brain.

40. See D. Sullivan, *Cosmetic Surgery: The Cutting Edge of Commercial Medicine in America* (New Brunswick, N. J.: Rutgers University Press, 2001).

41. See E. Showalter, *Hystories: Hysterical Epidemics and Modern Culture* (New York: Columbia University Press, 1997), and S. Hesse-Biber, *Am I Thin Enough Yet? The Cult of Thinness and the Commercialization of Identity* (New York: Oxford University Press, 1996).

42. See A. Rafalovich, "Exploring Clinician Uncertainty in the Diagnosis and Treatment of Attention Deficit Hyperactivity Disorder," *Sociology of Health and Illness* 3 (April 27, 2005): 305–323; I. Singh, "Doing Their Jobs: Mothering with Ritalin in a Culture of Mother Blame," *Social Science and Medicine* 59 (September 2004): 1193–1205; J. Leo, "American Preschoolers on Ritalin," *Society* 39 (January–February 2002): 52–60; R. DeGrandpre, *Ritalin Nation: Rapid-Fire Culture and the Transformation of Human Consciousness* (New York: W. W. Norton, 2000); J. Haber, *ADHD: The Great Misdiagnosis* (Lanham, Md.: Taylor Trade Publishing, 2003).

43. For a highly critical analysis of the increasing use of psychiatric medications among children, see J. Sparks and B. Duncan, "The Ethics and Science of Medicating Children," *Ethical Human Psychology and Psychiatry* 6 (Spring 2004): 25–39. See also J. Zito et al., "Trends in Prescribing of Psychotropic Medications to Preschoolers," *Journal of the American Medical*

Association 238 (2000): 1025–1030; M. Olfson et al., "National Trends in the Use of Psychotropic Medications by Children, *Journal of the American Academy of Child and Adolescent Psychiatry* 41 (2002): 514–521.

44. F. Fukuyama, *Our Posthuman Future: Consequences of the Biotechnology Revolution* (New York: Picador, 2002), pp. 54, 51–52.

45. The term "preemptive biology" was suggested to me by William Yoels, Professor Emeritus at the University of Alabama, Birmingham.

46. Healy, *The Creation of Pharmacology,* p. 355.

47. T. Szasz, *Ideology and Insanity* (Garden City, N.Y.: Anchor Books, 1970); R. Laing, *The Politics of Experience* (New York: Ballantine Books, 1967); E. Goffman, *Asylums: Essays on the Social Situations of Mental Patients and Other Inmates* (Garden City, N.Y.: Doubleday Anchor, 1961).

48. Horwitz, *Creating Mental Illness,* p. 130.

49. J. Hobson and J. Leonard, *Out of Its Mind: Psychiatry in Crisis— A Call for Reform* (Cambridge, Mass.: Perseus, 2002), p. 130. In addition, see Jerry Avorn's intelligent and balanced assessment of drug use in America entitled *Powerful Medicines* (New York: Knopf, 2004). Avorn argues that we need to do a better job assessing the benefits, risks, and financial costs of all drugs. "Used appropriately," medicines have great value. However, as he attests, we need to ask: "Just what is appropriate use? How can we know when the good outweighs the harm? And what is a reasonable cost to pay for this balance?" (p. 18). Common sense suggests that costly and powerful drugs are being misused when they are promiscuously prescribed to many who suffer merely from the normal vicissitudes of living.

Appendix A

1. Although the emergence of postmodern and feminist theories, in particular, have challenged the traditional social science canon of objectivity and the possibility of discovering fundamental and absolute social "truths," the dominant methodological paradigm in sociology remains committed to showing causal relationships through quantitative analysis of survey research data. A sampling of books that challenge the hegemony of the strictly scientific paradigm would include P. Collins, *Black Feminist Thought: Knowledge, Conscious-*

ness, and the Politics of Empowerment, 2nd ed. (New York: Routledge, 2000); S. Krieger, *Social Sciences and the Self* (New Brunswick, N.J.: Rutgers University Press, 1991); S. Harding, ed., *The Feminist Standpoint Theory Reader: Intellectual and Political Controversies* (New York: Routledge, 2004); C. Ellis and A. Bochner, eds., *Ethnographically Speaking: Autoethnography, Literature, and Aesthetics* (Walnut Creek, Calif.: Altimira Press, 2002); N. Denzin and Y. Lincoln, eds., *Handbook of Qualitative Research* (Thousand Oaks, Calif.: Sage Publishing Company, 2000).

2. The notion of allowing the world to "speak back" comes from H. Blumer, *Symbolic Interaction: Perspective and Method* (Englewood Cliffs: N.J.: Prentice Hall, 1969).

3. See B. Glaser and A. Strauss, *The Discovery of Grounded Theory: Strategies for Qualitative Research* (Chicago: Aldine Publishing Company, 1967).

4. R. Lewontin, "Sex, Lies, and Social Science," *New York Review of Books* (April 20, 1995), p. 29.

5. The phrase "better than well" comes originally from P. Kramer, *Listening to Prozac* (New York: Viking, 1993). See also C. Elliott, *Better Than Well: American Medicine Meets the American Dream* (New York: W. W. Norton, 2003).

6. See the appendix in C. W. Mills's book *The Sociological Imagination* (New York: Oxford University Press, 1959), entitled "On Intellectual Craftsmanship."

7. S. Andreski, *Social Sciences as Sorcery* (New York: St. Martin's Press, 1972), p. 108.

Acknowledgments

There is an intimate connection between my own life and the accounts of the fifty people I interviewed for this book. Each person helped me think more deeply about my own experiences with medication. For this reason I am very grateful to those who so freely shared their difficult and often heroic experiences. Social science stories must be absolutely grounded in respondents' feelings, thoughts, and observations. Their experiences constitute the core of this enterprise. I hope I have done justice to their words.

For nearly four years this book was the central activity of my life. Books consume their authors. Work that begins upon waking, dominates your thinking during the day, continues well into the evening, and typically follows you to bed inevitably finds its way into conversations with family, friends, colleagues, students, acquaintances, and even strangers. I am deeply grateful for the help of those who listened to me as I conceived this project, gathered data, shared my ideas about plausible lines of analysis, and completed the writing. Their comments and kindness influenced just how this book—this story—took shape.

It is a wonderful combination when colleagues are also good friends. For decades two of my colleagues at Boston College, Charlie Derber and John Williamson, have provided great friendship, terrific talk, wise ideas, and un-stinting encouragement. They are among the first to hear about new ideas and then about the inevitable periods of intellectual confusion and emotional uncertainty. We celebrate our birthdays together, commiserate endlessly about life's great challenges, muse about the state of the world, and mutually provide the kind of support neces-sary to complete projects requiring delayed gratification. The third member of my friend/colleague triad is Bill Yoels. Bill and I have collaborated on several books and articles. After a thirty-five-year working relationship, we pretty well know each other's intellectual moves. I have profited greatly from Bill's insatiable curiosity, prodi-gious scholarship, and honest criticism. Every time we talk I can count on a belly laugh or two and fresh insights that push along my thinking.

My editor at Harvard University Press, Elizabeth Knoll, got me quickly out of the starting gate through her sheer enthusiasm for this project. She has also helped guide the direction and content of this book. Among other things, Elizabeth persuaded me to include a separate chapter on the medication experiences of teenagers. Her careful read-ing of my pages, her many insights, and her gentle criti-cism surely made this a better book. She has also helped me become a better writer.

I am very fortunate to teach at Boston College for sev-eral reasons. First, the Sociology Department provides a sense of community that nourishes scholarship. Sec-ond, the university has consistently supported my work through grants to cover the cost of tape transcription, thus maximizing the time I can spend reading, thinking about the data, and writing. I am particularly grateful to my departmental chairperson, Stephen Pfohl, and to university administrators who arranged a sabbatical that allowed me to work full time on the book at a critical stage in its development. Third, I have the good fortune to work with unusually talented students at Boston College.

Lara Birk and I coauthored a paper that solidified my thinking for Chapter 4 of this book. Melissa Cox, Kelly Iwanaga, Mary Kovaks, and Molly Redding transcribed tapes at different stages of the interviewing process and offered valuable commentary on themes in the materials. Abigail Brooks, one of my graduate students, provided many thought-provoking conversations about drugs and personal authenticity. I also want to thank the students in two of my undergraduate classes. In an honors seminar titled "Important Readings in Sociology" and in an advanced undergraduate elective, "The Sociology of Mental Health and Illness," I got the chance to try out many of the themes central to the work. I am also grateful to Kate McManus and Michelle Carpentieri, who read preliminary chapters and provided gracious support and valuable feedback. This project was so encompassing that I even struggled to explain my ideas during French lessons with Brigitte Nicolas. I thank her for tolerating my clumsy French and for her insights into American medicine.

Finding adolescents to interview for Chapter 6 was a formidable exercise. I would not have been able to connect with young people without the help of Rina Cavallini and the Worcester, Massachusetts, branch of PAL (the Parent Professional Advocacy League), Dr. Barry Walsh and Kristen Danker of the G. Stanley Hall School, and Dr. Donald Zall, a therapist in the Boston area. As with all my writing on mental health issues, I am indebted to the MDDA support group (Manic Depressive and Depressive Association) that meets weekly at McLean's Hospital in Belmont, Massachusetts. MDDA's interest in and help with my work has always been more than I could hope for.

My greatest debt is to my wife, Darleen. More than anyone else she hears about the ups and downs that define the research and writing process. She has learned to navigate with great sensitivity the always-delicate spousal task of being both supportive and honest. Whether rearranging her schedule so that I might get to an interview, accompanying me on speaking engagements, reading draft chapters, or understanding the long hours spent in front of my computer, Darleen has been the true champion of my work.

Index